# A Practical Approach to Interdisciplinary Complex Rehabilitation

T0195156

# A Practical Approach to Interdisciplinary Complex Rehabilitation

Edited by

## Cara Pelser, BSc, PGCert, DClinPsych, CPsychol, PGDip
Clinical Psychologist in Neuropsychology
Cheshire and Merseyside Rehabilitation Network
The Walton Centre NHS Foundation Trust
Liverpool, England

## Helen Banks, MBBS, MRCP
Consultant in Rehabilitation Medicine
Cheshire and Merseyside Rehabilitation Network
St Helens and Knowsley Teaching Hospitals NHS Trust
Liverpool, England

## Ganesh Bavikatte, MBBS, MD, FRCP, FEBPRM
Clinical Lead
Cheshire and Merseyside Rehabilitation Network
The Walton Centre NHS Foundation Trust
Liverpool, England

ELSEVIER

ISBN: 978-0-7020-8276-4

9  8  7  6  5  4  3  2  1

For Information on all Elsevier publications visit our website at
https://www.elsevier.com/books-and-journals

**Content Strategist:** Poppy Garraway
**Content Project Manager:** Arindam Banerjee
**Design:** Margaret Reid
**Marketing Manager:** Ed Major

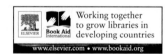

Working together
to grow libraries in
developing countries

www.elsevier.com • www.bookaid.org

Typeset by Aptara, New Delhi, India
Printed in Scotland

# Contents

## 4　Prolonged disorders of consciousness　　50
*Mary Ankers*

## 5　24-hour approach to physical management　　67
*Emily Wilson-Meredith and Emily Low*

## 6　Adjusting to life after illness or injury　　86
*Cara Pelser*

# Introduction

Cara Pelser, Angela Harrison, Helen Banks, and Ganesh Bavikatte

## Our hopes for this book

Pulling together firstly the authors, then determining the chapters and content, was not an easy feat. National Health Service (NHS) staff are incredibly busy people, throw a pandemic into the midst of author deadlines, and the challenge of creating a book worthy of publication becomes slightly stress-inducing, to say the least! As novel editors (well two of us, C.P. and H.B.), we hope that this book can support both the newcomer and the continuing professional development enthusiast, to understand the variety of roles present within the rehabilitation team, and how staff work together with patients and families to accomplish what is often unbelievable at the start of a patient's rehabilitation journey. Patients, following complex injury, illness or trauma, can present with a multitude of physical, emotional, behavioural, cognitive and psychosocial challenges, thus a dynamic team, who cross role boundaries, communicate, remain professional yet personable, and share a common goal (to optimise patient outcomes), can positively impact a patient's future. We hope that this book captures the passion and enthusiasm of all authors and that the reader will be encouraged by the notion that they too can add something significant to the field of specialist rehabilitation.

*A Practical Approach to Interdisciplinary Complex Rehabilitation* has been designed to introduce an integrated approach to the specialty of complex rehabilitation, organised into 15 chapters. The book provides a comprehensive, evidence-based, and practical guide to complex rehabilitation and interdisciplinary team (IDT) working. It covers all roles within the IDT to deliver a holistic approach to rehabilitation; including medical, nursing, dietetics, neuropsychiatry, occupational therapy, physiotherapy, psychology, rehabilitation coordination, speech and language therapy, and vocational rehabilitation therapy. The book is aimed at both current and aspiring health care professionals who are interested in the field of complex rehabilitation following injury or illness. It is one of the only books of its kind with a focus on each member of rehabilitation IDT, all in one place. In this way, important concepts of interdisciplinary working and the ethos of rehabilitation are reinforced. This was the inspiration for the book. To be truly interdisciplinary, you must engage in learning outside of your comfort zone, cross profession-specific boundaries, respect diverse ways of working and professional opinions, and ultimately consider the patient from a biopsychosocial perspective, whilst delivering patient-centred care (easy peasy, right?). Therefore, in a nutshell, this book is aimed at all who wish to learn more about the dynamic and diverse roles and responsibilities of the rehabilitation IDT who contribute to successful patient rehabilitation outcomes.

This book has been written by many authors, 25 to be exact, who are individuals with diverse skills and interests, and come from a variety of professional backgrounds and work across a range of settings from early acute rehabilitation to community rehabilitation. Therefore, each chapter is written in a style that is personal to the author/s, capturing further the diversity of the IDT. We have attempted to edit the book in a way that facilitates flow from one chapter to the next, however, the reader may choose to select chapters to read dependent on their current learning or special interest, their gaps in knowledge, or the time they have available for personal study.

We also hope that this book encourages personal reflection. The authors have each set out to write a chapter that facilitates reflective practice; a key skill in effective IDT working. Reflective practice amongst health care professionals ensures that we monitor our own actions and behaviours, develop self-awareness, and emotionally scrutinise our own beliefs, values, and moral compass, to ensure that we provide the best patient care we possibly can. Reflecting on the challenges, as well as the success stories, supports our learning and knowledge of the ever-expanding field of rehabilitation. With this evolution in mind, further reading is encouraged by each author, as the chapters within this book provide only a snapshot of the topic they set out to address.

## Where the idea for the book originated from

Back in 2017, the Cheshire and Merseyside Rehabilitation Network collaborated with Liverpool John Moores University to develop a 30 credit masters module titled 'Complex Rehabilitation in the Multidisciplinary Context', delivered by health care professionals working within the rehabilitation IDT. With the aim of sharing knowledge and expertise across disciplines and providing continuing professional development for staff who work in the field of complex rehabilitation, the module has now successfully been rolled out to neighbouring NHS Trusts and beyond. Given that the honorary lecturers had already planned PowerPoint slides, established reading lists, and delivered their specialist topics to keen students, a book which captured this incredible interdisciplinary working was identified as a side project, and deemed to be the next step in expanding and sharing knowledge.

The sharp-eyed observant reader will notice that the teaching module refers to multidisciplinary team (MDT) working and this book to IDT working. As discussed further in Chapter 1, MDT and IDT differ in their delivery of patient-centred care, with IDTs crossing professional boundaries when necessary and working more collaboratively, on a shared set of patient goals. The title of the book thus reflects the current ethos of the Cheshire and Merseyside Rehabilitation Network, its evolution from MDT to IDT working, and the inherently integrative nature of providing care across complex rehabilitation settings.

As one may imagine, early author (lecturer) discussions resulted in an increase in anxiety, worries that they 'didn't know enough' or 'didn't know where to start'. Uncertainty about what subject matter to cover in each chapter was expressed, and a lack of confidence in writing, and subsequently publishing was shared. Yet the busy authors embraced their inner imposter syndrome and like good (well great) NHS workers do they got on with the task at hand and developed, during a pandemic, a book to be proud of. We hope that you can take something meaningful from this book and transfer the key learning points which resonate with you into your everyday practice.

# Contributors

*Numbers in parentheses indicate the pages on which the authors' contributions begin.*

**Mary Ankers, (50)**, Advanced Clinical Specialist Speech and Language Therapist., Cheshire and Merseyside Rehabilitation Network, The Walton Centre NHS Foundation Trust, Liverpool

**Elaine Bailey, (164, 185)**, Advanced Clinician Speech and Language Therapist, Cheshire and Merseyside Rehabilitation Network, St Helens and Knowsley Teaching Hospitals NHS Trust, Liverpool

**Helen Banks, (18, xi, 258)**, Consultant in Rehabilitation Medicine, Cheshire and Merseyside Rehabilitation Network, St Helens and Knowsley Teaching Hospitals NHS Trust, Liverpool

**Lisa Barklin, (164, 185)**, Advanced Clinician Speech and Language Therapist, Cheshire and Merseyside Rehabilitation Network, St Helens and Knowsley Teaching Hospitals NHS Trust, Liverpool

**Ganesh Bavikatte, (18, xi, 258)**, Clinical Lead, Cheshire and Merseyside Rehabilitation Network, The Walton Centre NHS Foundation Trust, Liverpool

**Erin M. Beal, (242)**, Trainee Clinical Psychologist, Doctorate in Clinical Psychology Programme, Department of Primary Care and Mental Health, Institute of Population Health University of Liverpool, Mersey Care NHS Foundation Trust and University of Liverpool, Liverpool

**Nicola Branscombe, (137)**, Clinical Specialist Occupational Therapist, Cheshire and Merseyside Rehabilitation Network, The Walton Centre NHS Foundation Trust, Liverpool

**Antonio Swaraj DaCosta, (103)**, Consultant Neuropsychiatrist, Cheshire and Merseyside Rehabilitation Network, The Walton Centre NHS Foundation Trust, Liverpool

**Angela Harrison, (xi, 258)**, Performance, Information and Research Manager, Cheshire and Merseyside Rehabilitation Network, The Walton Centre NHS Foundation Trust, Liverpool

**Jo Haworth, (1)**, Clinical Specialist Physiotherapist, Cheshire and Merseyside Rehabilitation Network, The Walton Centre NHS Foundation Trust, Liverpool

**Claire Hendry, (242)**, Specialist Rehabilitation Nurse/Rehabilitation Coordinator, Cheshire and Merseyside Rehabilitation Network, The Walton Centre NHS Foundation Trust, Liverpool

**Nicola Hill, (39),** Specialist Rehabilitation Nurse/Rehabilitation Coordinator, Cheshire and Merseyside Rehabilitation Network, St Helens and Knowsley Teaching Hospitals NHS Trust, Liverpool

**Peter Kinsella, (119),** Principal Clinical Psychologist in Neuropsychology, Cheshire and Merseyside Rehabilitation Network, The Walton Centre NHS Foundation Trust, Liverpool

**Ray Langford, (222),** Occupational Therapist, Cheshire and Merseyside Rehabilitation Network, The Walton Centre NHS Foundation Trust, Liverpool

**Emily Low, (67),** Clinical Specialist Physiotherapist, Cheshire and Merseyside Rehabilitation Network, The Walton Centre NHS Foundation Trust, Liverpool

**Elly Milton, (235),** Expert patient, Liverpool

**Marie Milton, (235),** Expert family member, Liverpool

**Stephen Mullin, (137),** Consultant Clinical Neuropsychologist, Cheshire and Merseyside Rehabilitation Network, The Walton Centre NHS Foundation Trust, Liverpool

**Helen O'Leary, (1),** Physiotherapist/Rehabilitation Coordinator, Cheshire and Merseyside Rehabilitation Network, The Walton Centre NHS Foundation Trust, Liverpool

**Wendy Owen, (137),** Clinical Specialist Occupational Therapist, Cheshire and Merseyside Rehabilitation Network, The Walton Centre NHS Foundation Trust, Liverpool

**Cara Pelser, (86, 137, xi, 258),** Clinical Psychologist in Neuropsychology, Cheshire and Merseyside Rehabilitation Network, The Walton Centre NHS Foundation Trust, Liverpool

**Joanne Sim, (201),** Dietitian, Cheshire and Merseyside Rehabilitation Network, St Helens and Knowsley Teaching Hospitals NHS Trust, Liverpool

**Jon Alan Smith, (103),** Advanced Nurse Practitioner Neuropsychiatry, Cheshire and Merseyside Rehabilitation Network, The Walton Centre NHS Foundation Trust, Liverpool

**Rachel K. Taylor, (201),** Dietitian, Cheshire and Merseyside Rehabilitation Network, Liverpool University Hospitals NHS Foundation Trust, Liverpool

**Emily Wilson-Meredith, (67)**Physiotherapist, Cheshire and Merseyside Rehabilitation Network, The Walton Centre NHS Foundation Trust, Liverpool

# Acknowledgements

A novel project, of this size, required a tremendous amount of effort and contribution by many individuals. As editors, we would like to thank the wonderful authors who have dedicated so much time and effort to creating this book and to writing a chapter which reflects their understanding, experience and knowledge of complex rehabilitation. Two of the authors have personal experience of the rehabilitation network and interdisciplinary team working, and we would like to thank them both for sharing their personal narratives of being a patient/parent at the receiving end of care.

We would also like to thank Angela Harrison for her endless support, time and dedication to project managing the book behind the scenes. Without her, and her wonderful spreadsheets, we would have had no idea where each chapter was up to and the book would not have happened.

We would also like to thank the people who reviewed the proposal and those who took time to read over chapters and provide feedback to support the individual authors.

And lastly, a big thank you goes out to the support provided by Elsevier. It was difficult to write a book during a pandemic and yet we managed. Elsevier believed in our proposal and here we are with the final product!

Chapter 1

# Complex rehabilitation in an interdisciplinary team context

Jo Haworth and Helen O'Leary

## Chapter outline

### Abstract

To explore complex rehabilitation within an interdisciplinary team context and provide an understanding of how its concepts influence practice.

*Background/context*: Severe disabling illness or injury can result in a complex range of impairments and disabilities. Patients who present with complex illness or injury often require input from rehabilitation services. Complex rehabilitation has evolved considerably in recent years and it has become essential that health care professionals, whatever their discipline, have a deeper understanding of rehabilitation processes and rehabilitation pathways which will in turn allow the description and evaluation of effective rehabilitation interventions.

*Main ideas*: The following chapter will consider the important concepts underpinning rehabilitation practice. These will include the description of a framework which allows a common language to be used amongst health care professionals; models of care delivery, models of team working, and definitions of the rehabilitation pathway.

*Principal conclusions*: A return to the basic concepts, and a commitment to the application of these, will ensure that interdisciplinary teams keep the patient at the heart of their decisions and ensure that rehabilitation programmes are designed to be as effective as possible.

### Keywords

Complex illness; Complex rehabilitation; Maximise potential; Interdisciplinary teams

A Practical Approach to Interdisciplinary Complex Rehabilitation.
DOI: https://doi.org/10.1016/B978-0-7020-8276-4.00031-X

**1**

## Aim

To explore the concepts of an interdisciplinary team working within complex rehabilitation and how this influences practice.

## Objectives

- To describe and discuss the varied definitions of complex rehabilitation
- To understand how a framework for defining rehabilitation is useful in a clinical environment
- To examine the different models of team working in complex rehabilitation
- To identify the complex rehabilitation pathway
- To understand what 'Gold Standard' complex rehabilitation looks like

## Overview

By its very nature, severe disabling illness or injury can result in a complex range of impairments and disabilities. These may include physical, cognitive, emotional, social, and behavioural challenges for the individual. With such multifaceted care needs, patients who present with complex illness or injury often require input from rehabilitation services. A significant number of these patients may need prolonged involvement from specialist interdisciplinary teams with expertise in complex interventions (British Society of Rehabilitation Medicine (BSRM), 2014).

It has long been known by rehabilitation professionals that this type of specialist rehabilitation is a critical component of the care pathway, without which patient outcomes are likely to be compromised. Alongside extensive clinical backing, there is now a substantial body of evidence to support the clinical and cost effectiveness of specialist rehabilitation (BSRM, 2014, 2015). Research shows that despite a patient's longer length of stay, the cost of providing early specialist rehabilitation for patients with complex needs is rapidly offset by longer-term savings in the cost of community care (Turner-Stokes et al., 2006, 2015; Turner-Stokes, 2004, 2007, 2008).

With compelling arguments to support its provision, complex rehabilitation has evolved considerably in recent years. Health care providers recognise the need for timely, coordinated, complex needs-based programmes of care, delivered by specialist, interdisciplinary teams. Design and delivery of complex rehabilitation programmes and services requires an in-depth understanding of the essential components that define them (Graham, 2013; Wessex Strategic Clinical Networks, 2019; BSRM, 2009).

The aim of this chapter is to introduce complex rehabilitation within a health care setting and to define its key components; this should enable the reader to reflect on their own clinical experiences and apply new knowledge accordingly. It is intended that the knowledge gained will provide a solid foundation for health care professionals, whatever their discipline, to describe and evaluate rehabilitation interventions, rehabilitation processes, and rehabilitation pathways.

**TABLE 1.1 Patient scenario, Peter Black.**

**Patient: Peter Black**

*Present condition*
29-year-old male involved in a road traffic accident described as car versus tree at speed.
Multiple trauma-related injuries are listed as follows:

1. Subdural hematoma left-sided frontal lobe requiring craniotomy and evacuation
2. Fractured left humerus requiring conservative management
3. Multiple rib fractures right and left sided
4. Left-sided hemopneumothorax
5. Left fractured femur requiring internal fixation
6. Left compound fractured tibia and fibula requiring below knee amputation
7. Right fractured tibia and fibula requiring internal fixation

*Past medical history*

1. Recent history of excess alcohol
2. Asthma

*Social history*

1. Lived with his wife until recent separation
2. Two children, aged 4 and 6 years
3. Works as a car mechanic

*Clinical pathway*
Peter Black was admitted to accident and emergency, stabilised, and transferred to an
intensive care unit. Once stable, he was admitted to a major trauma ward to continue
with the required medical interventions and then moved to an inpatient specialist
rehabilitation unit. On discharge he returned home to live with his family and was
supported by the community specialist rehabilitation team

Each of the key rehabilitation components described within this chapter is applicable to each of the specialist domains described in the subsequent chapters, and to all stages within the clinical pathway. The learning from this chapter is therefore highly transferrable and will allow the reader to develop the building blocks for critical understanding and evaluation of complex rehabilitation in many health care settings.

A patient scenario (patient Peter Black) is detailed in Table 1.1. This scenario will be used to assist with activities and reflective learning throughout the chapter.

## What do we mean by 'rehabilitation'?

To understand rehabilitation as a concept, it is first essential to understand and explore its definition. This may sound like a simple place to start, yet just examining the detail in the definition of rehabilitation, will likely leave any health care professional with more questions than answers.

The most unifaceted definition comes from the Oxford Dictionary, which states that 'rehabilitation' is:

*The ability to restore to a good condition or to restore for a new purpose.*

(Oxford Dictionary)

The key words to highlight here are 'restore' and 'good condition' or 'new purpose'. These words provide a simple starting point for a developing discussion surrounding what rehabilitation might or might not look like. Although this definition was not developed with health care in mind, there are obvious links to what should be the ultimate goal for all health care professionals; supporting and enabling patients to get back to full health, or as close to this as possible. If full health is not possible, the goal of rehabilitation should be to support the patient to understand and manage the changes which have occurred, as a result of injury or illness.

Following disabling illness or injury, recovery is not likely to be as straightforward as the Oxford Dictionary definition. Rehabilitation professionals therefore require a more representative definition which accurately highlights the complexities of rehabilitation as a process. The medical literature describes many varied definitions of rehabilitation, and in aiming to understand what lies at the heart of the 'perfect' definition, it is important to critically appraise each description, considering the strengths and weaknesses of each. As a reader, you are encouraged to review and critique the following definitions.

Rehabilitation is:

*A problem solving and educational process aimed at reducing the disability and handicap experienced by someone as a result of a disease, always within limitations imposed by available resources and by the underlying disease.*

(World Health Organization (WHO), 2017)

*A set of interventions designed to optimise functioning and reduce disability in individuals with health conditions in interaction with their environment.*

(WHO, 2017)

*A process aimed at increasing human capacity by allowing people with health conditions to achieve and maintain optimal functioning by improving health, increasing participation in life, and increasing economic productivity.*

(WHO, 2017)

*A process aimed at maximising peoples' ability to live, work, and learn to their best potential.*

(WHO, 2017)

These definitions are certainly not exhaustive, therefore the reader is encouraged to research and appraise alternatives, to challenge their own perception of what rehabilitation means to them, both personally and clinically.

Within the above-listed definitions, there are a variety of words and phrases which encourage deeper consideration of the concept of rehabilitation.

The emergent themes include:

1. Problem solving
2. Educational
3. Enabling, increasing, maximising
4. Independence, participation in life
5. Optimum, potential
6. Limitations

Consideration of what each of the themes offers to the definition, and ultimately to the delivery of rehabilitation, should be an important element of any health professional's rehabilitation development. As you can see, the majority of the themes are positive and optimistic about future outcomes; however, remaining realistic and addressing potential limitations are a necessary requirement of successful rehabilitation.

Most health professionals are likely to choose their careers to 'help and care for others', and therefore the phrases 'enabling', 'increasing', and 'maximising' will feel comfortable and easy to engage with. The idea of addressing 'limitations' may feel somewhat uncomfortable to consider, however, a patient's limitations are just as much a part of rehabilitation as the positive themes highlighted above. Both those receiving and those delivering rehabilitation need to consider and understand the realistic limitations before rehabilitation can be considered successful.

## A framework for defining rehabilitation

As we have seen above, there are many different definitions of rehabilitation available within the health care literature, and in considering the merits of each, it is recognised that no single definition is able to cover all aspects of the 'rehabilitation process'. The WHO has provided many of the definitions cited throughout the literature and is considered a leading body of expertise in this area; yet even they have turned to more elaborate classification tools to facilitate a comprehensive understanding of what rehabilitation really is.

In 2001 the WHO created a framework to improve understanding of the concept of health and health-related status. This is known as the 'International Classification of Functioning, Disability and Health (ICF)'. The ICF is a multipurpose classification tool that is intended for a wide range of uses in many different health-related sectors (WHO, 2019; Stucki et al., 2007).

The framework was designed to allow its user to describe and organise information on a person's functioning and disability, and to provide a standard language and conceptual basis for the definition and measurement of health and disability. The framework's primary objective is to provide a descriptive profile of an individual's pattern of functioning, disability and health.

According to the ICF, as functioning and disability are multidimensional concepts, it is necessary to understand the multiple dimensions that form

**TABLE 1.2 The ICF framework.**

| Positive descriptors | Negative descriptors |
|---|---|
| Diagnosis/health condition | |
| Body structures | Impairment |
| Activities | Activity limitations (disability) |
| Participation | Participation restrictions (handicap) |

the concepts and to consider their definitions. These dimensions are listed as follows:

1. Body functions: Physiological functions of body systems (including psychological functions).
2. Body structures: Anatomical parts of the body such as organs, limbs, and their components.
3. Impairments: Problems in body function or structure such as a significant deviation or loss.
4. Activity: The execution of a task or action by an individual.
5. Participation: Involvement in a life situation.
6. Activity limitations: Difficulties an individual may have in executing activities.
7. Participation restrictions: Problems an individual may experience within life situations.

(Stucki et al., 2007)

   Table 1.2 provides a simple pictorial aid which aligns the terminology within the framework. This provides the ideal starting point for health care professionals to consider a patient's presentation, a patient's needs, and the potential impact on a patient's lifestyle. Once all of the elements of the framework are understood by health care professionals, the ICF becomes an essential tool for working in the specialist field of rehabilitation. It provides common language, terms, and concepts, from which the interdisciplinary team can describe the complexities of their own clinical practice and collaborate on overlapping areas of clinical practice.

## Clinical application

For a long time, the most commonly used ICF terminology included impairment, disability, and handicap. Even today, a proportion of the literature uses the 'negative descriptors' to describe health care assessments. The move to utilising alternative 'positive' descriptors (body structures, activities, and participation) was aimed at directing the focus of the ICF framework towards positive reviews and enablement, rather than negative reviews that disabled. Rehabilitation must be viewed as a process or journey that looks at what is possible for the individual,

**TABLE 1.3** ICF framework elements and examples.

| | |
|---|---|
| *Body structures/impairments* | |
| Abnormalities directly caused by the health condition | 1. Reduced range of movement<br>2. Reduced muscle strength<br>3. Poor short-term memory<br>4. Poor problem solving<br>5. Altered swallow<br>6. Receptive dysphasia<br>7. Low in mood<br>8. Poor bladder control |
| *Activities* | |
| Limitations in activities should be considered as a consequence of body structure abnormality | 1. Difficulties with transfers<br>2. Difficulty with mobility<br>3. Difficulties with personal care<br>4. Unable to prepare a meal<br>5. Unable to eat a meal<br>6. Difficulties with communication<br>7. Incontinent of urine |
| *Participation* | |
| Limitations in participation should always be considered as a consequence of 'limitations in activities' and leading from 'body structure abnormality' | 1. Unable to take the bus to work due to mobility issues<br>2. Struggling to hold down parental role in family unit<br>3. Difficulty with going out and social integration, i.e., eating out<br>4. Difficulties with answering the telephone<br>5. Fearful of leaving house, agoraphobia |

rather than what is not possible, and therefore the reader is encouraged to become expert in describing rehabilitation processes according to its positive features.

The framework and its descriptors provide multiprofessional health care teams with a common language that is independent of their own areas of specialism. Each of the multidisciplined teams will have knowledge of their own clinical responsibilities, and it is essential that they use the ICF framework to assist them in understanding and communicating this knowledge with other health care professionals. When starting to utilise the framework, professionals often find the detail confusing. However, with experience and understanding, it can assist professionals to look beyond their area of expertise, communicate within an interdisciplinary team (IDT), and focus on functioning rather than the diagnosis or condition; thus moving away from seeing the individual as just another 'patient'.

Table 1.3 summarises the framework elements and provides examples for the reader to identify with. The examples utilised cover the range of presentations that will be seen across the wide variety of treating disciplines in a complex rehabilitation environment.

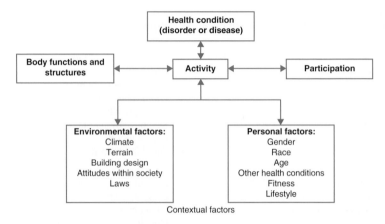

FIGURE 1.1    ICF framework, the reciprocal relationship.

Fig. 1.1 summarises the ICF framework again, but also provides evidence of the reciprocal relationships between body structures, activities, and participation. It introduces the reader to the contextual constructs described as environmental factors and personal factors. These factors are added into the framework to ensure that health care professionals are always focused on the individual. It may seem easier to consider and focus on the medical diagnosis or condition, according to the theory and knowledge we cover as an undergraduate, but this alone is not sufficient when working with people, who have individual minds, values, personalities, etc.

It is crucial to the success of rehabilitation that the health professional is aware of where a person has come from (their past personal experiences, health background and comorbidities, their mental health history, etc.), who they are now (cognitive, behavioural, social, physical factors, etc.) and where they are going to (their goals and aspirations). Rehabilitation must be individualised; therefore, the environmental and personal factors are a vital component of this framework.

Reflective questions

Consider the patient case study. What is Peter Black's health condition?

Describe Peter Black's possible body structure abnormalities (impairments), activity limitations, and participation restrictions.

What personal factors might influence Peter Black's presentation?

## Why is the ICF framework important to understand?

The ICF framework is relevant and effective when used for assessment and analysis across many health care settings. It can be applied to many contexts and at different levels starting from the single patient and their needs through to policy development, considering the needs of many.

These levels include:

1. The individual
2. The institution
3. Society
4. Economic analysis
5. Policy development
6. Research and interventional studies

(Barnes, 2003)

1. *The individual*
   This level relates directly to the patient and allows description of interventions that are designed and delivered to meet each patient's unique rehabilitation requirements. Here the framework can be used for:
   i. Detailed assessment of individuals
   ii. Person-centred treatment planning
   iii. Evaluation of the effectiveness of treatments and other interventions
   iv. Communication amongst IDT members
   v. Self-evaluation by patients

2. *The institution*
   This level relates to the overall rehabilitation programme/service provided to the patient. Here the framework can be used for:
   i. Education and training purposes
   ii. Resource planning and development
   iii. Quality improvement
   iv. Management and outcome evaluation
   v. Redesign within models of health care delivery

3. *Society*
   This level relates to how the abilities of a person, and the outcomes of a service, are then impacted by the environment and by societies values and perceptions. Here the framework can be used for:
   i. Eligibility criteria for entitlements and benefits
   ii. Social policy development, including legislative reviews, regulations, and guidelines
   iii. Complex needs assessments
   iv. Environmental assessment for identification of facilitators and barriers and implementation of mandated accessibility

4. *Economic analysis*
   This level relates to how the framework can assist with appropriate decision making for rehabilitation funding and commissioning choices. The ICF framework can enable the examination of whether resources are being efficiently used in health and social care settings. Within such examinations, it is important to weigh up the cost of people with functional limitations living

with support in the environment, against the cost of potentially changing the environment to allow them to live independently within it. Here the framework can be used to:

   i. Analyse the costs versus benefits of a variety of interventions and services

   ii. Direct the funding streams towards those interventions and services that evidence their effectiveness

5. *Policy development*

This level relates to how the framework can inform policy makers and legislative officials. People with complex health care needs accessing rehabilitation support are also service users, workforce members, and students within education. The ICF framework can be used to assist with providing population data which describe the impact of functional limitations, and informs policy development. Here the framework can be used to inform:

   i. Social security policy development

   ii. Employment law design and development

   iii. Education planning and support

   iv. Transportation needs assessments

6. *Research*

This level relates to how the framework is used as a tool to facilitate research design in rehabilitation. When evaluating research outcomes, the framework can allow comparison/synthesis of results by giving researchers a common focus. The evidence-based supporting rehabilitation is therefore strengthened as a consequence of synthesis and comparison of data. Here the framework can be used to:

   i. Facilitate research proposal design

   ii. Assist with appropriate outcome/objective measure choices

   iii. Allow comparison of research findings between studies and therefore consolidation of results

(Stucki et al., 2007)

**Reflective questions**

What might Peter Black's rehabilitation look like on his intensive care unit? What is Peter Black going to need from a rehabilitation unit, how could you describe his needs to potential commissioners? What might Peter Black's challenges be once he is living at home, how could you describe this to policy makers?

## Models of rehabilitation

Now that a clear definition and framework of 'rehabilitation' have been discussed, we will encourage the reader to explore how the elements of rehabilitation can be applied to clinical practice. We have examined how a person with complex illness or injury may present with limitations that impact on how they live their life, or considered from a different angle, how the way they live their life impacts on their limitations. This idea will be scrutinised further, as it is essential that rehabilitation professionals and teams pay attention to this when deciding how they will approach patient care.

There are various models of rehabilitation which may help inform this process:

1. *Medical model*: This model describes a person's activity limitations or participation restrictions as a direct result of their illness or injury. It assumes that these limitations or restrictions are 'problems' that the medical professional needs to treat and 'make better'.

2. *Social model*: This model describes a person's activity limitations or participation restrictions as a direct result of their social situation or environment. It assumes that if the social situation or environment were adaptable or more accommodating, the limitations and restrictions could have much less of an impact.

3. *Biopsychosocial model*: This model assumes that there are strengths within each of the previous models but that neither describes the most effective approach to rehabilitation. It describes a person's activity limitations or participation restrictions as needing both medical and social expertise and support. It requires a collaborative view of rehabilitation from patients, multidisciplinary teams, commissioners, and policy makers.

(Barnes, 2003; Wade and Halligan, 2017)

The biopsychosocial rehabilitation model is now quoted as the 'Gold Standard' for informing clinical interventions, outcome evaluation, pathway design, and social integration. Rehabilitation professionals should consider this model when designing packages of care, but they should also be ready to critically appraise its merits and suggest alternatives when challenged by their patient's needs.

**Reflective questions**

Describe the strengths and weaknesses of each model of rehabilitation. Consider under what circumstances and for what reasons each of the models might be the preferred choice within each of the stages of Peter Black's clinical pathway:

- Accident and emergency
- Intensive care
- Major trauma ward
- Inpatient rehabilitation unit
- Community team support at home

## Team working in rehabilitation

In clinical practice, a skilled workforce, represented by multiple disciplines, is essential to implementing an effective model of rehabilitation (WHO, 2019; National Health Service (NHS) England, 2016; Department of Health (DOH), 2005). It ensures that the full range of rehabilitation needs can be met, and that the multifaceted limitations faced by patients are addressed. The way in which a multiprofessional team works together and communicates in rehabilitation is vital in ensuring high-quality, efficient, and holistic care for patients (Barnes, 2003; Wade and Halligan, 2017). There are currently four recognised models for team working in rehabilitation, each of which has its strengths and weaknesses. A rehabilitation professional should understand these details and be able to describe which model works best in different situations. There are appropriate times and appropriate places for each of the models to be employed.

The four team working models are:

1. Unidisciplinary
2. Multidisciplinary
3. Interdisciplinary
4. Transdisciplinary

(Choi and Pak, 2006; NHS England, 2015)

1. *Unidisciplinary*
   Within this model, each professional team works independently of each other, working towards goals that are defined by their specific skills and experience. They are not often found collaborating on care, and work with other professionals only when required. See Fig. 1.2(A).
   Key elements:
   i. Professional focus on own interventions
   ii. Communication surrounding care tends to be between each professional team and the patient. It is not characterised by team collaboration
   iii. Works well when decisions need to be made quickly as it is easier to make them unilaterally
   iv. Tends to be seen in clinical areas where one particular profession is more dominant or has singular clinical responsibility
   v. Single discipline documentation/record
2. *Multidisciplinary*
   Within this model, each professional team works independently of each other, working towards goals defined by their specific skills, but there will be some collaboration on care and there will be some joint working and decision making. See Fig. 1.2(B).
   Key elements:
   i. Professional focus on own interventions
   ii. Communication surrounding care occurs between different disciplines and there is an emphasis on team collaboration
   iii. There will be formalised multidisciplinary team meetings
   iv. Multidisciplinary, joint documentation is expected, allowing a clear understanding of each other's assessments and interventions
3. *Interdisciplinary*
   Within this model, all of the professional teams work closely together often overlapping roles and clinical responsibilities. There will be a high level of

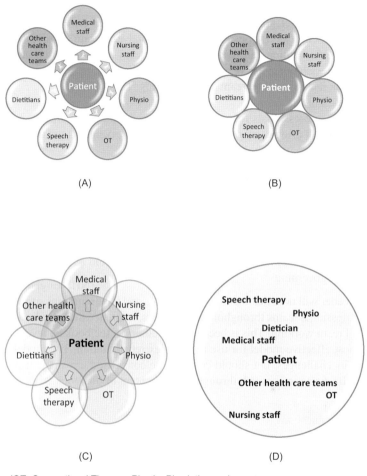

(OT, Occupational Therapy; Physio, Physiotherapy)

FIGURE 1.2    Model of multiprofessional team working. (A) Unidisciplinary team working. (B) Multidisciplinary team working. (C) Interdisciplinary team working. (D) Transdisciplinary team working.

collaboration on care and frequent joint working and decision making. See Fig. 1.2(C).

Key elements:

i.   Interprofessionals focus on team interventions

ii.  There is a high level of communication surrounding care between different disciplines, and a culture of team collaboration

iii. There will be formalised multidisciplinary team meetings and often cross discipline decision making

iv.  Multidisciplinary, joint documentation is expected showing clear evidence of collaborative assessments and interventions

4. *Transdisciplinary*
   Within this model, all of the professional teams work together, often blurring roles and clinical responsibilities. Traditional expectations of discipline-specific interventions are challenged, with team members often acting on behalf of each other. There will be a high level of collaboration on care, and decision making will be team driven. See Fig. 1.2(D).
   Key elements:
   i. Transprofessionals focus on team interventions means that team members will often carry out assessments and interventions not traditionally deemed to be within their remit
   ii. There is a high level of communication surrounding care and a culture of valuing all insights
   iii. There will be formalised multidisciplinary team meetings with cross discipline decision making
   iv. Multidisciplinary, joint documentation showing clear evidence of cross-boundary assessments and interventions
   v. The team members have equal accountability and as a result are often self-governing
   (NHS England, 2015)

   The reader will note that the title of this book, and all discussions surrounding multiprofessional teams throughout the chapters, reference the interdisciplinary model of team working. This is because the authors of the book believe that this is the most effective model for use in complex rehabilitation. The model is not without its challenges, but should certainly be considered a realistic aspiration and will be discussed as such throughout the content of this book.

Reflective questions

Describe the potential strengths and weaknesses of each team working model? Consider which model of team working might be the most effective within each of the stages of Peter Black's clinical pathway:
- Accident and emergency
- Intensive care unit
- Major trauma ward
- Inpatient rehabilitation unit
- Community team support at home

## The clinical rehabilitation pathway

All of the fundamentals discussed within this chapter thus far are essential when describing rehabilitation as a concept, but it is also important to consider at what point, in a health care pathway, rehabilitation is most relevant. This may seem a complex question requiring thought and discussion; however, the simple answer is that rehabilitation is both effective and necessary at all points along the pathway (NHS England, 2016; DOH, 2005).

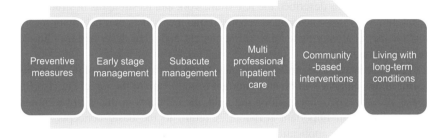

FIGURE 1.3   The rehabilitation continuum.

Interdisciplinary teams working within complex rehabilitation are encouraged to view the pathway as a continuum:

1. *Preventative measures*
   For example, health promotion
2. *Early stage management*
   For example, primary care teams, intensive care units
3. *Subacute management*
   For example, acute wards, specialist, or general
4. *Multiprofessional inpatient care*
   For example, hyper acute or complex rehabilitation units
5. *Community-based interventions*
   For example, community therapy services, primary care teams
6. *Living with long-term conditions*
   For example, education and self-management programmes

Fig. 1.3 summarises the rehabilitation pathway continuum.

Each section of rehabilitation already discussed, including definitions, frameworks, models of care, and team working descriptions, can be applied to each of the stages along the rehabilitation continuum. This will facilitate a deeper understanding of what 'care' should look like at each stage, and encourage health professionals to promote rehabilitation interventions at all points of the care pathway. Understandably, the involvement and interventions provided by health professionals vary, in terms of level and type, at each of the different stages, but there is one constant, and that is the patient themselves. The patient has been central to all rehabilitation elements discussed within this chapter, and should remain at the heart of the rehabilitation pathway.

## Summary

This chapter has presented an introduction to complex rehabilitation within an interdisciplinary team context. It has discussed a variety of definitions of rehabilitation and it has described the ICF framework and its strengths in structuring rehabilitation. It has encouraged debate around the models of rehabilitation care and the merits of varying team working models, and it has described the clinical rehabilitation pathway.

For those health care professionals new to rehabilitation, many of the concepts learnt in this chapter will be an important introduction to the topic, but also for those already experienced within the field, the concepts in this chapter should be considered an important revision. A return to the basic concepts, and a commitment to the application of these, will ensure that interdisciplinary teams keep the patient at the heart of their decisions and ensure that rehabilitation programmes are designed to be as effective as possible.

In the face of complex illness and injury presentations, it can be easy to forget what it is we are aiming for, why we do what we do, and crucially, who we are doing it for.

If we return to one of the definitions of rehabilitation from the beginning of the chapter, we should be aiming to:

'Maximise a person's abilities to allow them to live, work, and learn to their best potential' (WHO, 2017).

### Reflective questions

As you progress with the book, consider your learning from each individual chapter and aim to apply the concepts covered within this introduction. Ask yourself:

- How can I use the ICF framework?
- What model of care might be best utilised to deal with the issues?
- Which members of the team should be involved in the rehabilitation programme?
- What is the most effective way for each team member to work?

## References

Barnes, M.P., 2003. Principles of neurological rehabilitation. J. Neurol. Neurosurg. Psychiatry 74 (Suppl. IV), iv3–iv7.

British Society of Rehabilitation Medicine. 2009. British Society for Rehabilitation Medicine Standards for Rehabilitation Services mapped on to the National Service Framework for Long-Term Neurological Conditions. Available at: https://www.bsrm.org.uk/downloads/standardsmapping-final.pdf. Accessed September 18, 2019.

British Society of Rehabilitation Medicine. 2014. Rehabilitation for patients in the acute care pathway following severe disabling illness or injury: BSRM core standards for specialist rehabilitation. October 2014. Available at: https://www.bsrm.org.uk/downloads/specialist-rehabilitation-prescription-for-acute-care-28-11-2014-ja–(ap1-redrawn).pdf. Accessed September 18, 2019.

British Society of Rehabilitation Unit. 2015. Specialist neuro-rehabilitation services: providing for patients with complex rehabilitation needs. Available at: https://www.bsrm.org.uk/downloads/specialised-neurorehabilitation-service-standards–7-30-4-2015-pcatv2-forweb-11-5-16-annexe 2updatedmay2019.pdf. Accessed September 18, 2019.

Choi, B.C., Pak, A.W., 2006. Multi-disciplinary teams, inter-disciplinary teams and trans-disciplinary teams in health, research, services, education and policy: definition, objectives and evidence of effectiveness. Clin. Invest. Med. 6, 351–364.

Department of Health. 2005. National service framework for long-term conditions. Available at: www.gov.uk/government/uploads/system/uploads/attachment_data/file/198114/National_Service_Framework_for_Long_Term_Conditions. Accessed September 17, 2019.

Graham, L.A., 2013. Organization of rehabilitation services. Handb. Clin. Neurol. 110, 113–120.

NHS England. 2015. Multi-Disciplinary Team Development – Working Towards and Effective Multi-Disciplinary/Multi-Agency Teams. Available at: www.england.nhs.uk/wp-content/uploads/2015/01/mdt-dev-guid-flat-fin. Accessed September 17, 2019.

NHS England. 2016. Commissioning Guidance for Rehabilitation. Available at: www.england.nhs.uk/wp-content/uploads/2016/04/rehabilitation-comms-guid-16-17. Accessed September 17, 2019.

Stucki, G., Cieza, A., Melvin, J., 2007. The International Classification of Functioning, Disability and Health: a unifying model for the conceptual description of the rehabilitation strategy. J. Rehab. Med. 39, 279–285.

Turner-Stokes, L., 2004. The evidence for the cost-effectiveness of rehabilitation following acquired brain injury. Clin. Med. 4, 10–12.

Turner-Stokes, L., 2007. Cost-efficiency of longer-stay rehabilitation programmes: can they provide value for money? Brain Inj. 21, 1015–1021.

Turner-Stokes, L., 2008. Evidence for the effectiveness of multi-disciplinary rehabilitation following acquired brain injury: a synthesis of two systematic approaches. J. Rehab. Med. 40, 691–701.

Turner-Stokes, L., Pick, A., Nair, A., Disler, P.B., Wade, D.T., 2015. Multi-disciplinary rehabilitation for acquired brain injury in adults of working age. Cochrane Database Syst. Rev. 22, 12.

Turner-Stokes, L., Paul, S., Williams, H., 2006. Efficiency of specialist rehabilitation in reducing dependency and costs of continuing care for adults with complex acquired brain injuries. J. Neurol. Neurosurg. Psychiatry, 77, 634–639.

Wade, D.T., Halligan, P.W., 2017. The biopsychosocial model of illness: a model whose time has come. Clin. Rehab. 31 (8), 995–1004.

Wessex Strategic Clinical Networks. 2019. Rehabilitation is everyone's business: principles and expectations for good adult rehabilitation. Available at: www.networks.nhs.uk/nhs-networks/clinical-commissioning-community/documents/principlesandexpectations. Accessed September 16, 2019.

World Health Organization. 2017. Rehabilitation in Health Systems. Available at: www.who.int/rehabilitation/rehabilitation_health_systems/en/. Accessed September 17, 2019.

World Health Organization, 2019. International Classification of Functioning, Disability and Health (ICF). Available at: www.who.int/classifications/icf/en/. Accessed September 17, 2019.

# Chapter 2

# Medical management in rehabilitation

Helen Banks and Ganesh Bavikatte

## Chapter outline

## Abstract

This chapter identifies the crucial role of the doctor in the patient's recovery pathway. The role of the doctor in rehabilitation is often least understood/misunderstood by many, including clinicians. Specialist doctors usually take a lead role supporting patient and their loved ones, guiding the specialist team, and seeking appropriate external support when needed. Medical doctors hold the knowledge of the medical condition and likely recovery path and overall prognosis which is pivotal when setting specific, measurable, attainable, realistic, time-related (SMART) rehabilitation plans and long-term goals. The rehabilitation specialist doctor is able to monitor the rehabilitation progress, identify medical causes of disability, predict and proactively manage medical urgencies, and is able to provide the necessary help at different stages in the 'road to recovery'. The doctor not only plays a central role in symptom management and management of predictable or

A Practical Approach to Interdisciplinary Complex Rehabilitation.
DOI: https://doi.org/10.1016/B978-0-7020-8276-4.00002-3

unpredictable complications, but also acts as patients' advocate in their social and legal encounters.

**Keywords**
Specialist rehabilitation; Medical rehabilitation; Medical urgency in rehabilitation; Role of doctor in rehabilitation

## Aims

We hope that this chapter will support you to gain insight into the role of a rehabilitation specialist doctor.

The chapter has been subdivided to cover the following topics:

1. The role of the doctor within the specialist rehabilitation team.
2. Medical causes of complex disability.
3. The doctor's role in symptom management.
4. Medical urgencies commonly encountered during specialist rehabilitation.
5. The importance of understanding the diagnosis and prognosis.

Seven case examples have been included to illustrate the content of this chapter and to allow you to reflect on your learning.

## The role of the doctor within the specialist rehabilitation team

Rehabilitation is the process of helping an individual to achieve the highest level of function, independence, and quality of life after injury or illness (World Health Organization, 2001). This process supports and promotes any natural recovery, helps the patient to adapt to any residual impairment, and supports their family, friends, and carers.

Specialist rehabilitation is the total active care of patients with a disabling condition, by a multiprofessional team who have undergone recognised training in rehabilitation, led/supported by a consultant trained and accredited in rehabilitation medicine (British Society of Rehabilitation Medicine, 2015). The team works alongside the patient, family, and carers, taking a goal-orientated approach to address physical, cognitive, communication, emotional, financial, social, and vocational needs.

To become a consultant in rehabilitation medicine within the United Kingdom, a doctor will have commonly spent 5 years as a medical student, 2 years as a foundation doctor, 2–3 years as a core trainee (either in general medicine, general practice, surgery, or psychiatry) and 4 years in speciality training (traditionally rotating through neurorehabilitation, spinal injuries, amputee medicine, and musculoskeletal medicine).

A rehabilitation consultant leads the rehabilitation team. To do so, they need to assimilate a good, broad understanding of the skills and interventions offered by their interdisciplinary team colleagues. Using this, alongside their medical knowledge of disease processes, they can undertake thorough assessment of patients' rehabilitation needs and potential.

A rehabilitation doctor manages the rehabilitation patients' medical issues. They can manage medical instability and may support tracheostomy weaning. They support the management of a patient's underlying condition, and will address any general medical issues occurring during the process of rehabilitation. This may require liaison with other specialists, most commonly intensivists, trauma, acute care teams, and specialist medics and surgeons. Rehabilitation doctors have specialist skills in symptom management, including pain, bladder and bowel dysfunction, low mood, drooling of saliva (sialorrhea), and spasticity. They have in-depth knowledge of the potential complications of a patient's disabling condition and will support the management of such complications where preventive measures have been unsuccessful.

A rehabilitation doctor provides holistic care and will support emotional, social, vocational, and financial issues, often acting as an advisor and advocate for their patients.

## Medical causes of complex disability

Patients requiring specialist interdisciplinary rehabilitation will have complex disability with impairment of their physical, communication, cognitive or emotional abilities. Impairment could be a result of any individual injury/illness, or it could be due to a combination of conditions. Rehabilitation doctors are specialists in the approach to rehabilitation after illness or injury rather than in the diagnosis or management of specific medical conditions. However, there are groups of conditions that are more likely to lead to complex disability and are therefore seen more frequently within specialist rehabilitation. Rehabilitation doctors have enhanced expertise and knowledge of the conditions they see most often, which include:

1. Acquired brain injuries
2. Spinal injuries
3. Other neurological conditions
4. Polytrauma and musculoskeletal problems
5. Amputation

Each of these conditions will now be explored in further detail.

### Acquired brain injury

The brain is a complex organ, controlling our ability to breathe, move, talk, swallow, think, and feel. It can be injured via a variety of mechanisms; an overview is provided in Table 2.1.

The different areas of the brain all have various functions, see Fig. 2.1. Damage to a particular area, known to control a specific function, may cause impairment of that function. For example, damage to the occipital lobe may result in visual impairment. Some causes of acquired brain injury are more

**TABLE 2.1** Causes of acquired brain injury.

| Class | Description | Examples |
| --- | --- | --- |
| Traumatic | Brain injury caused by the consequences of the application of external forces to the brain, e.g., impact with the floor during a fall, severe shake during a road traffic accident, penetration by a weapon | Contusions<br>Subdural haemorrhage<br>Extradural haemorrhage<br>Subarachnoid haemorrhage<br>Diffuse axonal injury<br>Penetrating injury |
| Vascular | When there is disruption to blood flow within the cerebral blood vessels, the parts of the brain not receiving adequate blood become damaged. The presence of blood within the brain damages underlying brain tissue | Stroke; infarct or haemorrhage<br>Subarachnoid haemorrhage<br>Arteriovenous malformation<br>Venous sinus thrombosis<br>Asphyxia |
| Hypoxic | Damage to parts of the brain caused by a lack of vital oxygen reaching it | Cardiorespiratory arrest<br>Prolonged hypoxia<br>Asphyxia |
| Tumour | Tumour within the brain causes damage to the area it occupies and can cause swelling and bleeding into surrounding brain tissue | Malignant or benign tumours |
| Infection | Local or generalised damage to the brain due to the presence of infection which can be bacterial, viral, fungal, or parasitic | Meningitis<br>Encephalitis<br>Cerebritis<br>Abscess |
| Toxic/metabolic | Certain chemicals/substances can damage the brain tissue. These may be exogenous (from outside the body) or endogenous (from within the body) and present in elevated or reduced levels compared to normal | Recreational drugs<br>Alcohol<br>Radiation treatment<br>Central pontine myelinolysis/ osmotic demyelination (sudden change in blood sodium levels)<br>Hypoglycaemia (low blood sugar levels) |
| Inflammatory | Inflammation of the nervous system | Vasculitis<br>Multiple sclerosis |
| Other | Obstruction to the flow of fluid within and around the brain | Hydrocephalus |

likely to cause localised effects, for example, stroke or abscess, and others may cause more widespread damage, for example, vasculitis or hypoxia. In practice, patients with acquired brain injury are likely to present with a combination of impairments, owing to the complexity of the brain, and a prolonged period of

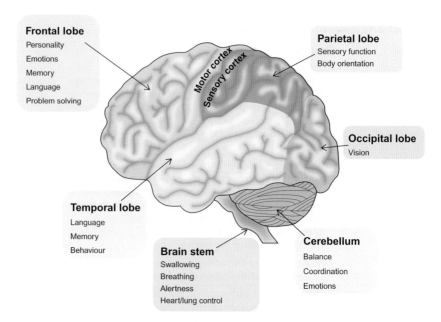

**Frontal lobe**
Personality
Emotions
Memory
Language
Problem solving

Motor cortex
Sensory cortex

**Parietal lobe**
Sensory function
Body orientation

**Occipital lobe**
Vision

**Temporal lobe**
Language
Memory
Behaviour

**Brain stem**
Swallowing
Breathing
Alertness
Heart/lung control

**Cerebellum**
Balance
Coordination
Emotions

FIGURE 2.1    Brain function diagram.

assessment may be required to identify these. For example, a patient presenting with a haemiparesis and dysphasia may also have cognitive and/or visual impairment that is not immediately apparent due to difficulty communicating their symptoms.

## Spinal cord injuries

The spinal cord plays a vital role in transmitting information between the brain and the body. It allows the brain to control movement of the trunk and limbs, the chest wall and diaphragm, and to empty the bladder and bowels. It sends sensory information from the body to the brain and is involved in the maintenance of blood pressure, body temperature, and supports sexual function and male fertility. The spinal cord is held within the 33 spinal vertebrae (the bones of the spine). At each vertebral level, peripheral nerves exit the cord to reach the proximal and distal parts of the body. The consequence of injury to the spinal cord depends on the level of injury and the part of the cord it involves.

American Spinal Injuries Association (ASIA, 2021) has developed the International Standards for Neurological Classification of Spinal Cord Injury which supports the detailed assessment of a spinal cord injured patient's motor and sensory responses. It helps teams to classify the injury and can be used to predict rehabilitation outcomes. For example, an Asia C6 type A injury describes an injury with no motor or sensory function below the sixth cervical level. The terms paraplegia, paraparesis, tetraplegia, and tetraparesis are also commonly used to describe levels and severity of impairment. 'Para' refers to the lower limbs only, 'tetra' to all four limbs, 'plegia' means complete loss of power, whilst 'paresis' refers to reduced power.

Causes of spinal injury include:

1. Trauma: road traffic accidents, sporting injuries, falls
2. Infection: discitis, epidural abscess
3. Inflammation: multiple sclerosis, transverse myelitis
4. Vascular: ischaemic, embolic or haemorrhagic events occurring within the spinal blood vessels
5. Tumour: benign, malignant, or metastatic
6. Degenerative (wear and tear) spinal conditions: movement of the vertebrae may cause compression of the spinal cord

Patients with complex spinal injury require a rehabilitation team with specialist skills. Rehabilitation doctors working within spinal cord injury are likely to have additional expertise in the management of respiratory dysfunction, neurogenic bladder and bowels, sexual dysfunction and dysautonomia (when the damaged spinal cord affects the body's ability to regulate blood pressure). They often support their patients lifelong, to reduce the risk of complications and guide them through life events such as pregnancy, surgery, and ageing.

## Other neurological conditions

Acute and chronic neurological conditions can result in complex disability. Many can cause acquired brain or spinal injury and have already been listed (Table 2.1). Others may affect the peripheral nerves (which transmit information between the skin, organs, and muscles to the spinal cord and brain) or directly affect the function of muscles. Those commonly seen in specialist rehabilitation settings include the following.

### Polyneuropathy

This group of conditions involves damage to multiple nerves, causes of which are many and include hereditary, toxic, inflammatory, and infections. Guillain–Barre syndrome is an inflammatory condition affecting multiple peripheral nerves (there are a number of variants). It often presents with ascending weakness and sensory disturbance (starts at toes and moves up the legs to the trunk, arms, and face) and may affect swallowing and respiratory muscles. Guillain–Barre syndrome can be a post-infectious phenomenon, following chest or gastrointestinal infections. Disability reaches a peak and then gradual recovery can be seen. This can take months, and a full recovery may not be reached.

### Spastic paraparesis

There are numerous conditions causing progressive weakness and spasticity of the lower limbs; these are often inherited, therefore running in families.

## Progressive conditions

Rehabilitation teams can help patients with conditions such as muscular dystrophy and motor neuron disease to optimise their current levels of function, adapt to disability and to plan for the future. Links with palliative care colleagues are invaluable when working with patients with life limiting conditions.

## Functional neurological syndrome

This presents with neurological symptoms which are not explained by disease. They may also be described as psychogenic, nonorganic, somatoform, dissociative, or conversion symptoms. The most common functional neurological symptoms are nonepileptic attacks and weakness, which are often mistaken for epilepsy or stroke. Functional symptoms often persist, and are associated with distress and disability (Stone, 2013). Our experience is that some patients with this condition respond well to interdisciplinary rehabilitation.

## Musculoskeletal conditions and trauma

Some specialist rehabilitation services are commissioned to work with patients with non-neurological illness or injury. This may include those with musculoskeletal injury or illness resulting in complex disability.

## Fractures and soft tissue injury

Causes commonly include falls, road traffic incidents, sporting accidents, or assault. Single or simple fractures are often rehabilitated within musculoskeletal/ orthopaedic services. Polytrauma (where there are multiple injuries) may lead to more complex disability and may also be associated with brain or spine injury and internal organ damage. Close links with trauma teams help to identify patients requiring specialist rehabilitation.

## Amputation

Rehabilitation after amputation is often managed on an outpatient basis by specialist limb loss and prosthetics services; however, where there is polytrauma or multiple limb amputation patients may benefit from inpatient specialist rehabilitation.

## Postural complications following immobility

Prolonged illness or immobility can be associated with the development of postural abnormality/contracture. For example, shortening of the soft tissues in the calf is seen commonly in those who have been bed-bound. This can lead to fixed plantar flexion of the feet and subsequent difficulty with standing or walking.

## Rheumatological conditions

With the development of disease modifying agents, those with rheumatological conditions have become less likely to develop complex disability and may not require specialist rehabilitation. However, some conditions remain highly disabling and links with rheumatology colleagues are important. Rheumatological disease as a comorbidity is often seen in specialist rehabilitation, for example, ankylosing spondylitis in those with spinal cord injury.

## The medics role in symptom management

Following injury or illness, a patient can present with a variety of symptoms and difficulties. These can be related to the type of illness or injury, the part of the body affected, the patient's emotional response, the provision of care and support, or they can be secondary to the medication or treatment used. Factors such as social support, home environment, finances, relationships, vocational and leisure activities, and patient expectations can all affect a patient's level of functioning following injury or illness. The rehabilitation doctor works alongside the interdisciplinary team to minimise the impact of symptoms after critical injury or illness. Commonly encountered symptoms and presentations are explored in detail below.

### Physical impairments

The most common physical symptoms the authors see in rehabilitation practice are spasticity, pain, bowel and bladder dysfunction, excessive drooling of saliva (sialorrhoea) and skin problems.

### Spasticity

Muscles affected by a brain or spinal injury can develop spasticity. This is a velocity dependent increase in tone, that is, the faster a spastic muscle is stretched, the tighter it becomes. Spasticity can be painful, can lead to postural deformities, and can interfere with functional activity. However, in some situations it can be helpful, for example, a weak leg may be supported in standing by increased tone within the extensor muscles.

Spasticity can be exacerbated by pain, infection, and stress; doctors need to explore and treat potential triggers in those presenting with worsening spasticity before treating the symptom itself. Spasticity can result in multiple complications, particularly when it is not identified or adequately managed. Spasticity can affect a patient's ability to walk, perform activities of daily living, sit, or sleep comfortably. It can contribute to the development of pressure ulcers or skin breakdown, contractures, and can cause pain. Following the development of spasticity, medical complications can develop as early as 4 weeks, and contractures can develop from 6 weeks. Spasticity may have an impact on every aspect of a patient's life. It is useful to consider the implications of spasticity using the framework of the WHO international classification of function, disability, and health (Bavikatte, 2017).

The management of spasticity should be undertaken by a coordinated multidisciplinary team, rather than by individual clinicians working in isolation

(Royal College of Physicians, 2018). Spasticity can respond well to a variety of treatments; the first line treatments are physical and include stretching and orthotic use. Medical treatments may be indicated as an adjunct to physical measures and include oral antispasmodic medication (e.g., baclofen, gabapentin, pregabalin, tizanidine, or dantrolene), intramuscular botulinum toxin, intrathecal treatments (baclofen or phenol delivered via the cerebrospinal fluid [CSF]) and surgical techniques (e.g., selective dorsal rhizotomy-cutting of sensory nerves to spastic muscles). Although often effective, medical treatments have the potential for side effects, and therefore must be carefully considered by the rehabilitation doctor when formulating a spasticity management plan with the patient and treating therapists.

---

**Case study 1: Asmita**

After a left-sided stroke, Asmita developed right-sided weakness and spasticity affecting her arm and leg. As a result, her right arm was held close into her body, her elbow held flexed (bent) and her fist clenched. She found it difficult to get her arm into her jacket, developed sores on her palm where her nails dug in, and was in pain when trying to get her splint on. In her leg, spasticity in her extensor muscles allowed her to straighten her leg and take her weight through it despite the weakness. Spasticity in her calf muscles caused her foot to point down and stopped her heel touching the floor when she was standing.

Medical treatment included baclofen tablets and botulinum injections to her right pectoralis muscle, elbow, wrist, and finger flexor muscles and her calf muscles (gastrocnemius and soleus). Alongside stretching and splinting, this proved beneficial, her heel was able to touch the floor which improved her gait, the sores on her palm healed, she was able to wear her splint, and she found dressing much easier.

Aside from doctors, which members of the interdisciplinary team may have helped Asmita with spasticity management?

---

## Pain

Patients with neurological injury or illness may experience altered sensation of the face, trunk, or limbs. This could be in the form of numbness, tingling/paraesthesia ('pins and needles') or neuropathic pain which is burning, shooting, or stabbing in nature.

Injuries to soft tissue, bones, and joints are likely to cause musculoskeletal pain which often throbs or aches. As those with neurological injuries are at risk of developing secondary bone, joint, or muscle problems, they can also present with musculoskeletal pain.

Pain can cause significant distress, impacting on sleep, mood and activity. This may form a vicious circle which can affect progress in rehabilitation.

The interdisciplinary rehabilitation team works together to improve a patient's experience of pain, and may use physical measures, psychological techniques and medical approaches to achieve this. Medical management may include the following:

1. Simple oral analgesics (paracetamol, ibuprofen)
2. Topical agents (lidocaine patches, capsaicin gel)
3. Oral neuropathic drugs (gabapentin, pregabalin, carbamazepine, amitriptyline, nortriptyline, duloxetine)
4. Opiates (codeine, morphine, fentanyl)
5. Nerve blocking injections, trigger point injections, or joint injections

Those with more complex pain, resistant to the above, may benefit from referral to specialist pain services.

## Swallowing and communication difficulties

Speech and language therapists take the lead in the assessment and management of communication and swallowing difficulties (refer to Chapter 11). Rehabilitation doctors may support this process, especially where pain, vomiting, presence of a tracheostomy, or poor saliva management exacerbates symptoms.

Drooling of saliva is a relatively common occurrence following a number of neurological insults; however, it remains under-recognised by clinicians as a problem. Even when recognised, it is often managed suboptimally. The proactive and multidisciplinary management of drooling can significantly improve the quality of life for patients and their carers (Bavikatte, 2017). Drooling of saliva occurs when patients are unable to swallow their own saliva effectively. This can be distressing for patients, irritate the skin (around the mouth, chin and neck, and chest) or lead to aspiration of saliva causing chest infections. Large volumes of saliva held within the mouth further impede verbal communication and swallowing. Rehabilitation doctors may prescribe medication to reduce the volume of saliva produced, which includes anticholinergic medications or botulinum toxin. Care needs to be taken to ensure the side effects of treatment are better tolerated than the symptom itself.

---

**Case study 2: Jason**

After a traumatic brain injury, Jason found it difficult to manage his own saliva. He had a tendency to drool, which he found embarrassing, and his voice often had a wet quality to it. He started using hyoscine patches (medication delivered via a sticky patch worn behind the ear) which helped reduce the drooling and improved his speech, however made him feel drowsy. The patches were discontinued and botulinum toxin was injected to his salivary glands instead. This also reduced drooling and improved the quality of his speech but without any side effects.

How else may this treatment have improved Jason's quality of life?

## Pressure sores

Those with reduced mobility are at risk of developing pressure sores. These are caused by the breakdown of skin and underlying tissue due to the application of prolonged pressure or shearing forces. They commonly occur at the sacrum, hips, heels, elbows, and occiput. The sore can be superficial or deep and can develop very quickly in those unable to self-relieve pressure. The presence of a pressure sore can affect a patient's ability to engage in the rehabilitation process and can take months to heal, commonly requiring specialist nursing input alongside medical care and dietetic support. Infection can develop within a sore and can spread to the underlying bone (osteomyelitis), which often requires prolonged courses of antibiotics to treat. Poorly healing sores may require surgical debridement and reconstruction. Prevention is the best treatment. Interdisciplinary working to optimise nutrition, hydration, and posture management and provide patient and carer education is vital.

## Bladder, bowel, and sexual dysfunction

Bladder and bowel dysfunction are seen commonly in rehabilitation settings and occur as a result of neurological damage, cognitive or emotional difficulties, reduced mobility, altered diet, and side effects from medications. This often presents with frequency, incontinence, or difficulty voiding urine and/or stool. Symptoms can be distressing, may affect a patient's engagement in rehabilitation, and can lead to increased care needs. A team approach to investigation and management is best, often with nurses and medics taking the lead. Urology and specialist bowel care teams may provide support in more complex cases. Investigations may include bladder diaries, blood tests, urinalysis, post void bladder scanning, X-ray, ultrasound, urodynamics (specialist test to assess bladder function), stool charts, stool analysis, bowel transit studies, rectal manometry (pressure measurement), and endoscopy (tube with camera inserted into bowel/bladder).

Treatment will depend on the cause. Bladder emptying may be optimised using simple techniques such as regular voiding, double voiding, or using a handheld bladder stimulator. Incomplete bladder emptying increases the risk of urinary infection, bladder stones and damage to the kidneys, and in cases not responsive to the above, intermittent self-catheterisation may be necessary. This requires the cognitive and physical ability to self-insert a urinary catheter, usually several times per day. Long-term catheterisation may be necessary if other management options are not successful.

Medication to reduce bladder irritability may help symptoms of urgency, frequency, and incontinence but can be associated with side effects including drowsiness and dizziness. Botulinum toxin to relax the bladder/urethra may also be helpful and is administered by the urology team.

Urinary incontinence not amenable to behavioural or medical measures may require the use of continence products including urethral/suprapubic catheters, sheath catheters, and continence pads/pants.

Constipation is commonly seen in patients following injury and illness. In severe cases this can lead to overflow diarrhoea, fecal impaction, and bowel obstruction. The early development of a bowel management routine is therefore essential and includes adequate hydration and nutrition, posture management, minimising the use of constipating medications and providing support to encourage the bowels to open regularly. This may be achieved simply with regular toileting (ideally sitting on toilet/commode rather than bedpan) or by taking advantage of the gastrocolic reflex which stimulates voiding after meals.

In neurological illness or injury, stool transit through the bowel may be slowed, placing the patient at high risk of constipation. Sensory and motor control of the anorectum may be impaired leaving the patient with reduced or absent voluntary control of the process of defaecation. This combination of impaired continence and risk of severe constipation is termed neurogenic bowel dysfunction (Multidisciplinary Association of Spinal Cord Injury Professionals, 2012). Careful assessment of the problem is required in order to provide appropriate management. Laxative medications may be prescribed to soften/bulk stools or to increase bowel motility. Abdominal massage and digital rectal stimulation may be used to encourage bowel movements. Suppositories or enemas may encourage stool to come away from the rectum. Some patients with severe bowel dysfunction may require long-term manual evacuation of stool performed by nurses/carers. Specialist bowel care teams may offer bowel irrigation when symptoms are resistant to more simple measures, or in some cases, the formation of a colostomy (bowel opens into a bag on abdomen).

Sexual dysfunction is common following injury and illness and can be caused by neurological damage, emotional distress, or side effects of medication. Sexual dysfunction can have a negative impact on a patient's mood and relationships, but concerns may not always be raised due to embarrassment or discomfort. A PLISSIT model (Annon, 1976) offers a succinct method for introducing sex into a clinical conversation and offering effective counselling and treatment. Its name derives from the four levels of intervention: permission, limited information, specific suggestions, and intensive therapy. Rehabilitation doctors should explore whether a patient has any concerns about sexual function and offer support where able to. This may involve review of medications (many can affect sexual function), management of other symptoms (e.g., pain and spasticity), use of medication for erectile dysfunction, signposting to support groups advice regarding sexual aids, or referral into specialist services such as urology, gynaecology, or sexual health services.

## Cognitive and behavioural difficulties

Cognitive and behavioural difficulties can occur as a result of damage to the brain, a pre-existing medical condition (e.g., dementia), concomitant mental health conditions, or as a result of medication/treatment, biochemical/hormone imbalance, hydrocephalus, or infection.

A rehabilitation doctor will consider the cause of cognitive or behavioural difficulties and investigate and treat as appropriate. They will review medications, aiming to withdraw, where possible, those known to exacerbate cognitive impairment or behavioural difficulties. They will work closely with the interdisciplinary team to optimise the patient's environment and identify and remove any triggers to challenging behaviour, however, they may need to offer medication to manage agitation. Medications can include benzodiazepines (sedatives), antipsychotics, and antiepileptics, all of which have potential side effects and should be reviewed regularly and withdrawn when possible.

---

**Case study 3: Dan**

Dan had moved to a rehabilitation unit following a traumatic brain injury. He had been started on olanzapine (antipsychotic) and sodium valproate (antiepileptic) for agitation early on during his acute admission. Occasional episodes of challenging behaviour were still seen, but agitation was significantly improved. Fatigue and cognitive difficulties were proving to be a barrier to his progress, with limited physical carryover from session to session and variability in his ability to engage. Different causes of fatigue were considered but investigations were all normal. It was felt that his medication might be contributing to fatigue, and olanzapine and sodium valproate were gradually withdrawn. After a few weeks his fatigue, engagement and progress within therapy sessions were seen to improve markedly.

Take a moment to think about what this case teaches us.

---

## Prolonged disorders of consciousness

This is discussed in detail within Chapter 4. Assessment of patients with reduced conscious level can be complex and takes time. It is very important to ensure that patients with the cognitive ability to interact and express themselves are supported to do so. The rehabilitation doctor will explore any additional causes of drowsiness or fatigue; for example, pituitary dysfunction leading to hormone imbalance, hydrocephalus, infection, anaemia, or medication side effects. At present there is insufficient evidence with respect to the use of medication to enhance arousal/awareness, although emerging evidence from recent trials suggests that at least some patients may benefit from amantadine during the recovery phase (Royal College of Physicians, 2020). Careful consideration is required before trialling medication to enhance arousal, and the patient's family and interdisciplinary team should be involved.

## Visual and hearing impairment

Visual loss, altered acuity, double vision, blurred vision, field loss, and visual neglect are commonly seen after brain injury. The rehabilitation doctor undertakes basic assessment of vision and works with the therapy team to understand the impact of visual problems on a patient's functional abilities. They will liaise with orthoptics and ophthalmology where further specialist investigation and management are required.

Problems with hearing can affect a patient's ability to communicate and follow instruction with subsequent impact on their rehabilitation. New problems may be related to a brain injury and specialist ENT review required. Simple issues such as wax build-up can be easily addressed.

## Emotional sequelae

All patients will experience emotional sequelae following their injury or illness which could include personality changes, mood swings, emotional lability, depression and anxiety, frustration and anger, sense of loss, post-traumatic stress disorder, and paranoia/psychosis. These could affect not only their participation and progress, but also their relationships and vocational opportunities. Rehabilitation doctors need to work alongside psychologists and psychiatrists to explore emotional issues and consider management, which may include the prescription of medication. Antidepressant medications are commonly used in rehabilitation settings, care needs to be taken when choosing an antidepressant as some are contraindicated in certain conditions or patient groups. Some antidepressants have additional therapeutic uses and can be used for dual purposes, for example, duloxetine is also used to manage neuropathic pain.

## Social, vocational, financial, and legal issues

Life changing illness or injury may affect a patient's social, financial, and legal situation. A rehabilitation doctor has a crucial role in providing medical information (with patients' consent) to outside agencies. They are often asked for reports and opinions to guide return to work/retirement applications, ongoing care needs, provision of benefits, and return to driving. They may also complete medicolegal work such as police witness reports, capacity assessments, applications for power of attorney, and as expert witnesses in court of protection cases.

## Medical urgencies encountered in specialist rehabilitation

Any acute medical, surgical, or psychiatric problem may present itself during rehabilitation, and initial care is provided by the rehabilitation doctor. Depending on the issue, the location, facilities of the unit, and the skill set of the team, the rehabilitation doctor will decide whether continued care can be provided in the rehabilitation setting, or, if transfer to acute services/other specialities is required. Patient safety is paramount. An unwell patient is unlikely to be able to participate actively in rehabilitation, and the priority should be optimal treatment of their acute illness.

Common urgent medical issues experienced by a patient undergoing rehabilitation can be categorised as follows:

1. Related to their injury/illness: for example, further brain haemorrhage or, infarction, hydrocephalus, sepsis, seizures, progression of pathology
2. Related to their disability: for example, aspiration pneumonia, pressure sores, thromboembolism
3. Related to comorbidities (other coexisting medical conditions): for example, ischaemic heart disease, gout, diabetic complications
4. Iatrogenic (as a result of treatment): for example, side effects from medication, feeding tube/catheter blockage, hospital acquired infections

The ABCDE approach (Resuscitation Council UK, 2016) is used by many when dealing with acute medical urgencies. This stands for Airways, Breathing, Circulation, Disability and Exposure and encourages the responder to take a safe and systematic approach to the assessment and management of the acutely unwell patient.

The following case studies will demonstrate the presentation of urgencies within rehabilitation and the diagnoses to be considered. Place yourself in the position of the rehabilitation doctor as you work through each case.

**Case study 4: Sarah**

Sarah, 55, is rehabilitating after a subarachnoid haemorrhage. This has resulted in moderate cognitive impairment, reduced balance, and mild right-sided weakness. She had been progressing well until the nurses notice she is drowsy and ask you to review her.

What do you think may have caused her drowsiness and how would you approach this situation?

Causes of Sarah's reduced conscious level could include:

1. Seizure
2. Further cerebral bleeding
3. Extension of stroke
4. Increased intracranial pressure
5. New traumatic brain injury
6. Hydrocephalus
7. Sepsis
8. Side effect of medication
9. Biochemical abnormality

You might take an ABCDE approach to assessment and management and then move on to a more detailed examination. More information about her condition and treatment can be found by reviewing notes and drug charts, observations and imaging, and through discussion with the treating nurses. Simple tests may include blood tests, blood sugar, arterial blood gases and urine analysis. Imaging such as X-rays, CT, or MRI may be required, and depending on the findings, specialist tests such as lumbar puncture and CSF analysis or electro encephalography may be indicated.

Treatment depends on the cause, some of which are discussed in more detail below.

## Sepsis

Sepsis is defined as life-threatening organ dysfunction caused by a dysregulated host response to infection (Singer, 2016). Within a rehabilitation setting, common sources of infection are chest, urine, central nervous system, or skin. Sepsis is a medical emergency. Investigations include bloods, cultures, and imaging. Treatment is according to the local sepsis protocol, antimicrobial prescribing guidelines and liaison with the microbiology team. Escalation to acute or critical care settings may be required.

## Seizure

A seizure is caused by sudden, uncontrolled electrical activity in the brain affecting movements, behaviour, feelings, and conscious levels. A focal seizure affects one part of the body, while a generalised seizure affects multiple parts of the body and reduces conscious levels. All require thorough assessment, investigation, and management. Prolonged generalised seizures can pose immediate risk to life.

A seizure can be precipitated by injury to the brain and can occur at the time of injury, shortly after injury or be delayed by weeks, months, or years. They can also be caused by primary epilepsy, alcohol withdrawal, and biochemical abnormalities.

Common investigations include blood tests, brain imaging, and electroencephalogram (which looks at the electrical activity within the brain). Medical treatment of an acute seizure is dictated by the local protocols; the underlying cause or trigger should be treated where possible and preventive antiepileptic medications may be required. Patient and family education is important to reduce risk of harm from future seizures.

## Hydrocephalus

Hydrocephalus can occur when there is a blockage to the flow of CSF within the brain, causing enlargement of the ventricles (fluid filled spaces) and subsequent compression of surrounding brain tissue. This blockage can be caused by bleeding, infection, or a lesion within the brain and can present soon after a brain injury or after a delay of weeks or months.

Hydrocephalus can manifest as headache, vomiting, and reduced conscious level, or if developed gradually, can show more subtle signs such as confusion, abnormal gait, and incontinence. Brain imaging and lumbar puncture can be used to confirm the diagnosis, and management is neurosurgical with controlled drainage via a catheter or shunt.

> **Case study 5: Luca**
>
> Luca, a 33-year-old gentleman, is new to the rehabilitation unit. He was involved in a road traffic accident and sustained a severe traumatic brain injury and multiple rib fractures. He has a tracheostomy in situ and his level of awareness is reduced. His respiratory rate has increased to 30 breaths per minute and the nurses ask you to review.
>
> How would you approach this case and what do you think could be causing his symptoms?

Again, the ABCDE approach will support you to assess and stabilise the patient. A detailed history and examination, review of notes, drug chart, and observations would be indicated. Arterial blood gases, electrocardiogram, blood tests, and a chest X-ray may be requested.

This gentleman is tachypnoeic (breathing fast). This symptom is seen in respiratory distress, with dysautonomia (both discussed below), and as a result of some metabolic conditions. Pain and anxiety can also cause a patient to breathe rapidly.

## Respiratory distress

Respiratory distress occurs when the lungs cannot meet the body's oxygen requirements. Thinking about Luca, causes of his respiratory distress could include:

1. Chest infection
2. Pulmonary embolism
3. Chest secretions can restrict the airways and could block a tracheostomy if severe
4. Weakened respiratory muscles mean more effort (faster breathing) is required to meet his oxygen requirements
5. Traumatic pneumothorax (presence of air in the pleural space between the lung and its lining) which compresses the lung.
6. He may have been given too much intravenous fluid causing pulmonary oedema (fluid on the lungs)
7. He may be asthmatic, have a cardiac condition, or have another chronic lung disease

As with all medical urgencies, management would depend on the cause. If oxygen levels are low, supplementary oxygen may be required whilst investigation is undertaken. Severe respiratory distress may require intensive care support and ventilation.

## Dysautonomia

Dysautonomia occurs when the autonomic nervous system does not function optimally. This may affect the functioning of the heart, bladder, intestines, sweat glands, pupils, and blood vessels.

In some patients, severe injury to the parts of the brain regulating autonomic function can cause dysautonomia (also called sympathetic storm or paroxysmal sympathetic hyperactivity). This consists of periodic episodes of increased heart rate and blood pressure, sweating, hyperthermia, and motor posturing, often in response to external stimuli (Meyfroidt, 2017). These symptoms mimic other medical urgencies and can often be mistaken for sepsis. Medical treatment including beta-blockers, gabapentin, pregabalin, opiates, and benzodiazepines may help.

Autonomic dysfunction can also be seen in those with spinal cord injury; here it presents differently and is called autonomic dysreflexia and is more common in those with injuries affecting the thoracic or cervical spinal cord. Triggers including urinary retention, constipation, sexual activity, labour, pressure ulcers, soft tissue injury, fractures, burns, ingrown toenail, and menstrual cramps prompt an overactive sympathetic response. The most prominent component of autonomic dysreflexia is a dramatic rise in blood pressure (Bycroft, 2005). Patients may also have headache, an intense feeling of anxiety, vasodilation (with sweating, warmth, redness) above the level of spinal cord injury, vasoconstriction (with goose bumps, coolness, pallor) below the level of injury, chest tightness, bradycardia (slowed heart rate), and dilated pupils. Untreated this can cause seizures, brain haemorrhage, and coma. Urgent identification and removal of the trigger is the most effective management, and medication to reduce blood pressure may be used in the interim and depend on local policy.

## Prognosis

A realistic prediction of outcome is essential in order to plan the rehabilitation programme, support patients and their families to adjust to life after injury and illness, and to allow early identification of longer term care needs, environmental adaptations and support services. A rehabilitation doctor needs to take a holistic approach when considering prognosis, and consider the patient factors, rehabilitation factors, and external factors at play.

### Patient factors

A rehabilitation doctor will need to use their knowledge and experience of the medical condition when formulating a prognosis. Some conditions offer a good prognosis for recovery, others are variable, and some are progressive, suggesting further deterioration will be seen with time. Although the medical diagnosis plays a crucial role, the doctor also needs to consider a patient's comorbidities, age, cognitive abilities, emotional state, support network, and social situation, as these will also have an impact on their recovery and overall outcome.

**Case study 6: Ana**

Ana suffered a severe traumatic brain injury at the age of 23, requiring surgical intervention, critical care, inpatient, and community rehabilitation. There was initial doubt with regard to her potential to survive her injuries; however, within 2 months she was starting to walk with therapists. She had significant cognitive deficits and was intermittently agitated. Over the course of the next 3 months she made considerable improvements within activities of daily living and was discharged to her parents' home with residual fatigue and moderate cognitive impairment. After 6 months of community rehabilitation she was managing well in her own home, and after a further year, she had returned to full-time education.

What factors do you think may have influenced Ana's recovery?

## Rehabilitation factors

Service-related issues can influence a patient's outcome and may relate to the expertise and availability of the rehabilitation team, the provision of rehabilitation equipment, or the rehabilitation teams' links with other specialities and agencies. Patients can benefit from peer support which is dependent on their ability to interact with other patients during their rehabilitation. Infection control measures can limit some patient's access to group work, equipment, and social opportunities, which may impact on their rehabilitation.

## External factors

The availability of quality community care, appropriate equipment, technology, and environmental adaptations can vary depending on a patient's locality, their financial situation or their diagnosis. This can also influence outcome.

It is important to remember that every patient is unique and no two patients with the same injury/illness will follow the same course. Whilst patients can exceed expectations, they can also struggle to meet goals. Continued support for the patient, family, and team is required during rehabilitation, with regular review and adjustment of goals in accordance with the progress of the patient and the expectations of the team.

**Case study 7: Henry**

Henry is an 85-year-old gentleman who was previously well with no significant comorbidities. He suffered a right-sided stroke with resultant left-sided weakness and dysphagia. The stroke team felt he had rehab potential beyond the provision of their service and he was transferred to a level 2 specialist rehabilitation unit. He spent 3 months undertaking an intensive rehabilitation programme. Goals included progressing to oral diet from gastrostomy feeding, using a standing method for transfers, and achieving functional use of the left arm. Within individual therapy sessions, progress was seen; however, fatigue was marked and the intensive therapy required to progress abilities in one area seemed to have a knock-on effect on another; progress to supported standing prompted optimism from the team, however was followed by several days of severe fatigue and a deterioration in his swallowing ability. Alterations to his timetable and intensity of therapy were made, but no overall functional gains were seen. He was discharged home with equipment for transfers and a package of care, taking some diet orally but still required the gastrostomy tube to meet his nutritional needs.

Consider the impact of this case from the perspective of; Henry and his family, the interdisciplinary team members, and the rehabilitation service.

## Summary

Please take a moment to reflect on this chapter. What knowledge can you take away with you and apply to your day-to-day role?

Within this chapter we have covered some of the more commonly encountered diagnoses seen within specialist rehabilitation, discussed how the doctor may support in symptom management, and described some of the urgent complications rehabilitation patients may experience. If you would like to read more about any of the topics we have touched upon, the references below may guide your further reading.

In the United Kingdom, rehabilitation medicine is a small speciality which is poorly understood by nonrehabilitation doctors, allied health care professionals, health care managers, and the general public, and there is an assumption that therapists alone direct rehabilitation. We hope this chapter has described the important and varied role of the specialist rehabilitation doctor, and their position as an integral interdisciplinary team member.

## References

American Spinal Injury Association, 2021. International Standards for Neurological Classification of SCI (ISNCSCI) Worksheet - American Spinal Injury Association. Available at: https://asia-spinalinjury.org/international-standards-neurological-classification-sci-isncsci-worksheet/. Accessed October 27, 2021.

Annon, J.S., 1976. Behavioural Treatment of Sexual Problems: Brief Therapy. Harper & Row, Oxford, England.

Bavikatte, G., et al., 2017. Spasticity Work Book: Early and Ongoing Management. Common Patterns, Botulinum Toxin Treatment, Ultrasound Localisation, Post-treatment Exercises. Ganesh Bavikatte, United Kingdom.

British Society of Rehabilitation Medicine, 2015. Specialist neuro-rehabilitation services: providing for patients with complex rehabilitation needs. Available at: https://www.bsrm.org.uk/downloads/specialised-neurorehabilitation-service-standards–7-30-4-2015-forweb.pdf. Accessed October 27, 2021.

Bycroft, J., et al., 2005. Autonomic dysreflexia: a medical emergency. Postgrad. Med. J. 81 (954), 232–235.

Meyfroidt, G., et al., 2017. Paroxysmal sympathetic hyperactivity: the storm after acute brain injury. Lancet Neurol. 16 (9), 721–729.

Multidisciplinary Association of Spinal Cord Injury Professionals, Guidelines for Management of Neurogenic Bowel Dysfunction in Individuals With Central Neurological Conditions, 2012.

Resuscitation Council UK, 2016. Advance Life Support Manual, seventh ed.

Royal College of Physicians, 2018. Spasticity in adults: management using botulinum toxin. National guidelines. Available at: https://www.rcplondon.ac.uk/guidelines-policy/spasticity-adults-management-using-botulinum-toxin. Accessed October 27, 2021.

Royal College of Physicians, 2020. Prolonged disorders of consciousness following sudden onset brain injury: national clinical guidelines. https://www.rcplondon.ac.uk/guidelines-policy/prolonged-disorders-consciousness-following-sudden-onset-brain-injury-national-clinical-guidelines. Accessed October 27, 2021.

Singer, M., et al., 2016. The third international consensus definitions for sepsis and septic shock (Sepsis-3). JAMA 315 (8), 801–810.

Stone, J., 2013. Functional neurological symptoms. Clin. Med. (Lond.) (1) 80–83.

World Health Organization, 2001. International Classification of Functioning, Disability and Health: ICF. WHO, Geneva.

## Chapter 3

# The role, impact, and reflections of the rehabilitation nurse

Nicola Hill

## Chapter outline

### Abstract

The aims of this chapter are to provide an introduction to the role of a rehabilitation nurse and to explore the importance and impact of this specialty. It is hoped these insights will encourage the reader to think about this unique role, carried out in various settings, and the positive impact the rehabilitation nurse has, not only in the direct care of patients and families/carers, who experience some of the most traumatic and life-changing events, but also crucially, within the interdisciplinary team, and wider community. The chapter provides opportunities for the reader to think about the qualities and skills of the rehabilitation nurse, and reflect on both the challenges and rewards of nursing within this specialist field, hopefully raising its profile amongst others who work or are interested in the field.

### Keywords

Rehabilitation nursing; Responsibilities; Roles; Family and carer support; Nursing goals; Discharge; Community

## Aims

1. To provide an introduction to the role, qualities, and skills of the rehabilitation nurse.

A Practical Approach to Interdisciplinary Complex Rehabilitation.
DOI: https://doi.org/10.1016/B978-0-7020-8276-4.00003-5
**39**

2. To explore the importance and impact of rehabilitation nursing with the patient and their family.
3. To reflect on the challenges and rewards of this specialty.
4. To raise the profile of rehabilitation nursing as an integral role within the complex rehabilitation interdisciplinary team.

## Introduction

Rehabilitation nurses work in various settings, including hospitals, inpatient rehabilitation centres, long-term care facilities, and within community services. They work with patients who are often going through the most vulnerable and traumatic times of their lives. A review of the literature fails to define the role of the rehabilitation nurse within the United Kingdom. Despite the importance of nurses in rehabilitation being highlighted since 1980, it appears that little progress has been made towards raising the profile of this nursing specialty (Jester, 2007). In comparison, when exploring the literature internationally (predominantly from the United States of America, Canada, and Australia), clear definitions of the role of the rehabilitation nurse can be found, and there is a sense of the rehabilitation nurse being truly recognised and embedded within rehabilitation services.

This chapter will support the reader to gain insight into the role and impact of the nurse within complex rehabilitation. This will be partly self-reflective, drawing on my personal experiences as a rehabilitation nurse, but we must acknowledge that each nursing role is multifaceted and unique in nature, requiring a variety of skills and qualities. This chapter will also seek to explore how the rehabilitation nurse can positively impact not only the patients under their direct care, but also the wider rehabilitation team, carers, and families.

It is hoped that with increased insight into the role and opportunities within rehabilitation nursing, those readers with nursing backgrounds may consider a career in this field, and that those outside of nursing will use it to further develop their own interdisciplinary approach to patient care. There is opportunity at the conclusion of each section for the reader to reflect on their own thoughts or practice.

## Definition, roles, and responsibilities of a rehabilitation nurse

A rehabilitation nurse will 'assist individuals with a disability and/or chronic illness to attain and maintain maximum function' and in 'adapting to an altered lifestyle, while providing a therapeutic environment for client's and their family's development' (The Association of Rehabilitation Nurses, 2015).

Patients who have experienced a major traumatic illness or injury require nurses who are able to provide care and treatment within complex situations whilst maintaining a person-centred approach. There are a number of conditions/diagnoses that may result in the need for complex rehabilitation (these are explored further in Chapter 2), nurses will need to be familiar with these and be able to provide crisis interventions and specialist assessments/treatments alongside the standard nursing care activities.

As many patients have comorbidities, an essential part of rehabilitation nursing is to support both the disabling condition and any other chronic condition, which may also cause some level of impairment and deconditioning.

The roles and responsibilities of the rehabilitation nurse can be thought of as clinical and nonclinical (Table 3.1). Describing these will hopefully go some way to demonstrating the breadth of expertise and knowledge that can be gained from a career within rehabilitation nursing.

### Reflective questions

Taking into account what you have read so far, what do you think are the challenges and rewards of rehabilitation nursing?

## Family and carer support

Aadal et al.'s (2017) work explored the perceived role of the nurse in an inpatient stroke setting and reported that the 'nurses expressed that they have a threefold purpose; to take care of the patient, to take care of the relatives, and to support the interaction between the patient and relatives'. Sadly, a recent Headway study in the United Kingdom established that out of those caring for a patient with a brain injury (British Society of Rehabilitation Medicine, 2009):

- 60% felt they do not receive adequate support in their caring duties.
- Only a quarter had received a carer's assessment.
- Half were not aware that they were entitled to a carer's assessment, despite the legal requirement for local authorities to ensure carers are made aware of their right to assessment.
- 18% rate their quality of life as poor or very poor.
- 59% show signs of clinical depression with 21% in the severe or extremely severe range.

Furthermore, Barber (2018) states 'if the physical, social and mental health needs of caregivers are not addressed by healthcare professionals, they are likely to have a serious and significant impact upon the physical, social and mental wellbeing of the patient'. According to State of Caring (2010), 'A new duty is required by the NHS in England, Wales and Northern Ireland to put in place policies to identify carers and promote their health and wellbeing'. Due to the holistic nature of complex rehabilitation and the length of time patients are known to a service, rehabilitation nurses are well placed to identify carers requiring support and to signpost to local services.

**TABLE 3.1 The roles and responsibilities of the rehabilitation nurse.**

| Clinical | Nonclinical |
|---|---|
| Respiratory management:<br>Including tracheostomy care and weaning, secretion management<br>Optimising skin integrity:<br>Managing wounds, burns and grafts<br>Stump care<br>Providing bespoke care to prevent the development of pressure sores<br>Developing bowel and bladder management plans:<br>Assessment and identification of dysfunction<br>Providing support and education on management techniques such as bladder retraining, intermittent self catheterisation, bowel irrigation and provision of manual evacuation<br>Correct use of manual handling equipment and specialist equipment:<br>This includes specialist seating<br>Demonstrating use of equipment for family and carers<br>Supporting enteral and parenteral feeding and modified diets:<br>This requires closely working with dietetics, SLT and catering teams as well as families and carers<br>Spasticity and contracture prevention and management:<br>Applying splints and braces correctly<br>Care of patients before, during, and after treatments such as botulinum toxin injections, intrathecal baclofen pumps, tendon lengthening procedures<br>Supporting pain management:<br>Administering medication, assessing pain scores, and providing a holistic approach to pain management | Act as a role model and mentor for patients, nursing staff and students:<br>This may include a keyworking or named-nurse role (in which consistency and continuity of care for an allocated number of patients are provided) and acts as a single point of contact for patients and families or carers<br>Promote the improvement of nursing care and rehabilitation nursing<br>Educate patients, families, and carers by:<br>Promoting patient and family or carer adaptation and adjustment to lifestyle changes<br>Apply nursing research to clinical practice to ensure evidence-based practice care is delivered<br>Contribute to a safe, therapeutic, and enriching environment by:<br>Undertaking risk assessments, audit and service improvement projects<br>Engage with local governance policy<br>Participate in activities that will positively influence the community's awareness of disabilities<br>Identify person-centred nursing goals by:<br>Being adaptable and able to meet the needs of patients with a variety of conditions and diagnoses, and co-morbidities through continued learning and self-development<br>Assist with social re-integration<br>Co-ordinate a holistic approach to meeting patient needs:<br>Identify leisure activities,<br>Peer support services,<br>Charitable organisations<br>Complex discharge planning activities<br>Liaison with other specialties and services |

*(continued on next page)*

**TABLE 3.1 The roles and responsibilities of the rehabilitation nurse—cont'd**

| Clinical | Nonclinical |
|---|---|
| Providing safe environment for expression of psychological needs and time for listening: Supporting challenging behaviour Identifying triggers (or antecedents) and patterns, working with the IDT to put supportive strategies in place | Contribute to goal planning, in interdisciplinary (IDT) meetings and discharge planning meetings Represent the IDT out of working hours, by being able to provide patients, and their families or carers with updates pertaining to nursing and to other disciplines, and take forward any queries or concerns |
| Fatigue management and pacing activities to ensure adequate rest and sleep | |
| Identifying and exploring sexual health needs | |
| Medication management: Education and monitoring Supporting patients to progress to self-administration of medication | |
| Providing access to spiritual care | |
| Supporting patients with cognitive and communication impairments: May need to use strategies or communication aids Competently undertake capacity assessments and work within legal frameworks to safeguard the vulnerable | |
| Advocate on behalf of patients | |
| Supporting assessment of patients with Prolonged Disorders of Consciousness (PDOC): This can present with its own ethical dilemmas for the rehabilitation nursing teams This subject will be covered in more depth in chapter 4 | |

It is vital to ensure that family/carers are actively involved in goal planning/discharge planning meetings, facilitating home leave, and supporting their loved one in their rehabilitation journey and beyond. Nurses are well placed to take the lead in communicating with carers/family as they are likely to be around at visiting time when issues can be explored, updates can be delivered, and a rapport can be developed. Chapter 15 will discuss how the socioeconomic needs of patients and their carers can be supported.

## Formulating nursing goals and assessing outcomes

Some nurses may not be familiar with the concept of setting SMART (Specific, Measurable, Achievable, Relevant, Timed) goals, and have not been provided with the opportunity to gain experience in goal setting for patients in the same way as our Allied Health Professional counterparts are. However, the traditional nursing process is transferable and lends itself to this concept. Many nursing models have independence and holistic care at their core (Jester, 2007). Using this knowledge, goals can be set specifically with a nursing focus or, ideally, collaboratively with other disciplines. This would encourage patients to view their rehabilitation as not just the formal therapy sessions with separate disciplines, but as a more continuous and seamless process.

Rehabilitation nurses are constantly working towards goals with their patients which can easily be made SMART and incorporated into the goal planning process, examples include:

- Self-management of pressure relief whilst in wheelchair.
- Increase nutritional or fluid intake.
- Increase mobility outside of formal therapy sessions.
- Increase independence within grooming tasks, washing and dressing activities.
- Applying own brace/splints.
- Decreasing pain levels by introducing self-medication.
- Reducing incontinence using bowel and bladder routines.

The UK Specialist Rehabilitation Outcomes Collaborative collates data nationally for patients with highly complex needs accessing multidisciplinary, specialised rehabilitation (NHS Commissioning Board, 2013). Several of the outcome measures collected are used to assess patients' levels of dependency and record the specialist interventions provided. Rehabilitation nurses have a key role in providing this information and are likely to be involved in completing:

1. Functional Independence Measure + Functional Assessment Measure: The UK Functional Independence Measure + Functional Assessment Measure assessment tool is a global measure of disability for the brain injured population. It is the mandatory outcome measure for level 1 and 2 specialist rehabilitation units.
2. Rehabilitation Complexity Scale.
3. NPDS (Northwick Park Dependency Score) is a nursing specific indicator. NPDS has been shown to be valid, reliable, and practical to use. It was designed to be used together with a short set of additional questions to inform care needs in the community and facilitate discharge planning. The NPDS can be utilised to set goals for patients and to monitor their progress. The tool can be effective in predicting care needs for individuals but also for groups of patients within the complex rehabilitation setting.

These nursing sensitive outcome measures can also be used for reviewing staff establishment and commissioning arrangements. The data collated can be utilised to reflect the complexity and changing needs of the service and its users and stakeholders.

It is also recognised that there may also be nursing indicators and risk assessments that are required locally, within each rehabilitation environment, whether it be inpatient or community.

**Reflective questions**

Take a moment to think about a patient you have seen recently and develop a SMART nursing goal.

## Caring for patients with reduced mental capacity

Decisions about care and treatment for patients who lack capacity in England are governed by the Mental Capacity Act (2005). Nurses in all adult care settings need to be familiar with the relevant legislature within the country they practice. The aim of this section is not to discuss how mental capacity assessments are carried out, or to guide the reader through the complex arena of Deprivation of Liberty Safeguards. Instead, this section will briefly note the decisions which need to be carefully explored and considered by the nursing and wider interdisciplinary team. Further, more detailed reading is recommended for the rehabilitation nurse, who plays a crucial role in mental capacity and ensuring that patients, under their care, are protected and empowered. Further information on mental capacity is provided in Chapter 7 and Chapter 10.

The assessment of a patient's capacity to consent is commonly required within rehabilitation settings, especially when working with patients following acquired brain injuries. Examples of decisions to be considered include:

- Admission to the unit
- Level of nursing observation, provision of supplementary care
- Falls prevention strategies/equipment
- Use of wheelchair belts, bed rails, and bed tables
- Refusal of treatment/care
- Administration of covert medication
- Discharge planning decisions
- Use of the internet and social media
- Need for modified diet
- Financial support and decisions
- Engagement in sexual activity

If a patient does not have the mental capacity to make a decision for themselves, a best interest's decision may be required. This may necessitate a formal meeting with relevant members of the interdisciplinary team, family, carers, and outside agencies.

Rehabilitation nurses need to have up-to-date knowledge of legislation and local policies, they need to be aware of all mental capacity issues and any best interest decisions affecting the patients under their care. They need to be aware of any advanced directives, lasting power of attorney or court of protection orders involving their patients, and act in accordance with the law.

**Reflective questions**

Take a moment to think about one of the decisions listed above and how a rehabilitation nurse may approach the mental capacity assessment.

## Discharge planning

Following completion of a specialist inpatient rehabilitation programme, many patients will require complex discharge planning. This requires careful consideration of their environment, equipment, and care needs, alongside their social and financial situation. An effective and safe discharge can be achieved by:

- Working closely with the patient and their family/carers.
- Interdisciplinary team working with assessments for specialist equipment, home and/or environmental visits.
- Identification of care needs and planning for community provision.
- Trials of home leave or use of independent living units (requiring nurses to mimic community care packages)
- Referral for onwards community therapy.
- Referral for community nursing care: district nurses, tissue viability nurses, community matrons, community rehab nurses, continence teams.
- Forging close links with third sector agencies and groups.
- Developing and awareness of charitable organisations and community groups.
- Safeguarding patients who may be vulnerable, undertaking mental capacity assessments.

A rehabilitation nurse may be responsible for coordinating discharge and will need to possess a working knowledge of the support services and funding streams available locally. In the United Kingdom, funding streams may include health care funding, social care funding, private income, charitable or litigation funds.

## Community rehabilitation nurse

As discussed previously, there is limited literature available in the UK field of rehabilitation in regard to the unique role of the nurse. This is also found to be true in the area of community rehabilitation nursing. The Association of Rehabilitation Nurses from the United States (2018) provides insight into the role of the homecare rehabilitation nurse. This is deemed as essential in the continuity of care. Furthermore, the role is also cost-effective, whilst still providing specialist knowledge and skills. In collaboration with the rest of the multidisciplinary team, the homecare rehabilitation nurse continues to function as a clinical resource, a care coordinator, an advocate, a primary care provider, a teacher, a consultant, and a team member, centred around patient-driven goals (Association of Rehabilitation Nurses, 2018).

Within the Cheshire and Merseyside Rehabilitation Network, there is a rehabilitation coordination team. The role of the rehabilitation coordinator can be fulfilled by health care professionals with the relevant skills and experience, coming from various disciplines including nursing. Each rehabilitation coordinator is a key contact for patients and families or carers during the patient's rehabilitation journey, from admission to discharge, and into the community. The coordinator provides advice to patient and families and carers and addresses any questions or concerns. They are an integral part of the interdisciplinary team and possess a variety of experience and skills, depending on their clinical background.

The rehabilitation coordinators assess new referrals for complex inpatient or community rehabilitation, presenting their findings and opinion back to the consultant and coordination team. They organise the weekly IDT meetings to discuss patients care, treatment, and progress. They are instrumental in keeping patients, families, and carers informed and involved throughout the inpatient rehabilitation journey, the patient is in the right setting at the right time. They also help to prepare for rehabilitation beyond hospital discharge and into the community and provide information about professionals and agencies who can provide ongoing support and help.

---

### Case study: David

At this stage in the chapter, considering a case study from the perspective of a rehabilitation nurse may help to consolidate understanding of the role. Please read through the case and consider the questions posed.

David, a 45-year-old man, was admitted to a major trauma ward following a road traffic accident. He had a learning disability and worked part time at a local garden centre. One of his siblings was his main source of support.

David sustained the following injuries:

- Thoracic spinal fractures
- Multiple rib fractures

(continued)

**Case study: David — cont'd**
- Bilateral pneumothoraces and pulmonary contusions
- Fractured left humerus (upper arm) requiring surgical fixation
- Grade 1 splenic lacerations
- Open fracture left tibia, fibular (lower leg) requiring surgical fixation
- Left transtibial (below knee) amputation
- Cerebral haemorrhage and contusions (bruising to the brain)

David was intubated and required surgical tracheostomy. He spent 1 month in a neurological intensive care unit. He had a slow respiratory wean.

What would the nurse's role be at this stage of David's rehabilitation?

David was transferred to a hyperacute rehabilitation ward, with a tracheostomy in situ (cuffed). Following decannulation of his tracheostomy, he was transferred to a level 1 complex rehabilitation unit in order to continue his rehabilitation journey.

David was in 'Post-Traumatic Amnesia' for about 4 weeks following his injury. He had neurological deficits which included impaired vision, sensory impairment, dysphagia, cognitive difficulties, and agitation.

What do you think the rehabilitation nurse's goals and role would be at this level of David's rehabilitation?

Following 3 months at the level 1 unit, David was admitted to a level 2 rehabilitation unit. He required assistance from two members of staff with all his care needs and was using a hoist for all his transfers. He was able to engage with staff and some carryover was evident.

What do you think the nurses' goals and role would be at this level of David's rehabilitation?

Six months later, at discharge, David required supervision at all times to prevent falls. He was taking normal diet and fluids. He was able to maintain his sitting posture, transfer with assistance, and walk short distances with a wheeled Zimmer frame. He had mild residual cognitive impairments and some agitation.

David was referred to a specialist community rehabilitation team, local authority Social Work Learning Disability Team, and local District Nursing team.

Is there a role for a community rehabilitation nurse to support David moving forward?

## Development of the rehabilitation nurse role

Rehabilitation nurses may wish to develop further specialist skills to progress their careers within rehabilitation, this may include, for example, continence care, pain management, or wound care.

Other opportunities may also present themselves to a nurse with rehabilitation skills and experience. Examples may include:

- Advanced practitioner or specialist nurse in a speciality, such as trauma, head injury, or stroke.

- Rehabilitation coordinator, within inpatient, community, or extended rehabilitation service.
- Senior nurse or ward manager, matron of a rehabilitation service.
- Research nurse.

## Summary

- Nurses have an integral role in rehabilitation within the interdisciplinary team, providing 24-hour care to patients, working towards the best outcomes for each individual.
- The rehabilitation nursing role is varied, requiring a combination of skills and a holistic approach to patient care.
- Rehabilitation nurses also provide support to patients, families, and carers.
- It is imperative that nurses recognise the value that they possess in the rehabilitation process, in order to promote this to the wider team that they work with.
- Further recognition of the role of the rehabilitation nurse is required in order to raise the profile of the specialty.
- Rehabilitation nursing provides good opportunity for career progression.

## References

Aadal, L., Angel, S., Langhorn, L., Pedersen, B.B., Dreyer, P., 2017. Nursing roles and functions addressing relative during in-hospital rehabilitation following stroke. Care needs and involvement. Scand. J. Caring Sci. 32 (2), 871–879.

Association of Rehabilitation Nurses Position Statement, 2015. Rehabilitation Nurses Play a Variety of Roles. Availiable at: https://rehabnurse.org/about/roles-of-the-rehab-nurse. Accessed January 6, 2021.

Association of Rehabilitation Nurses Position Statement, 2018. What Does a Home Care Rehabilitation Nurse Do. Available at: https://rehabnurse.org/about/roles/home-care-rehabilitation-nurse. Accessed January 6, 2021.

Barber, C, 2018. Working with informal caregivers: advice for nurses. Br. J. Nurs. 27 (19), 1104–1105.

British Society of Rehabilitation Medicine, 2009. British Society for Rehabilitation Medicine Standards for Rehabilitation Services mapped on to the National Service Framework for Long-Term Neurological Conditions. Available at: https://www.bsrm.org.uk/downloads/standardsmappingfinal.pdf. Accessed September 18, 2019.

Jester, R., 2007. Advanced Practice in Rehabilitation Nursing. Blackwell, Oxford, p. 8.

Mental Capacity Act, 2005. Available at: https://www.legislation.gov.uk/ukpga/2005/9/contents. Accessed September 30, 2021.

NHS England, NHS Commissioning Board, 2013. NHS Standard Contract for Specialised Rehabilitation for Patients With Highly Complex Needs (All Ages). Available at: https://www.england.nhs.uk/wp-content/uploads/2014/04/d02-rehab-pat-high-needs-0414.pdf. Accessed December 16, 2020.

State of Caring, 2010. A snapshot of unpaid care in the UK, Available at: https://carersuk.org/stateofcaring. Accessed September 30, 2021.

## Chapter 4

# Prolonged disorders of consciousness

Mary Ankers

## Chapter outline

### Abstract

With advances in acute medical and trauma care, rehabilitation teams are recognising an increasing number of patients surviving severe acquired brain injury but presenting in a prolonged disorder of consciousness (PDOC). This chapter identifies the key interdisciplinary practices that are required when caring for individuals in a vegetative state or minimally conscious state. Current PDOC guidelines and research findings are considered in the context of a pathway model of rehabilitation. Challenges in diagnosis and the potential for misdiagnosis of PDOC are considered from an interdisciplinary perspective. However, clinical diagnosis neither determines what is in a patient's best interests nor how their rehabilitation pathway is structured. Person-centred approaches to PDOC care and rehabilitation—which incorporate family and friends as key partners—are described. Findings from functional magnetic resonance imaging and sEMG studies challenge our view of consciousness and how it is assessed in a clinical context. Interdisciplinary teams must keep best interests considerations front and centre, as they balance diagnostic information from clinical assessments and emerging novel research tools. It is recognised that clinicians in this area may be working in extended scope roles and require specific support for professional development and wellbeing.

### Keywords

Prolonged disorders of consciousness (PDOC); Vegetative state (VS); Minimally conscious state (MCS); Best interests

A Practical Approach to Interdisciplinary Complex Rehabilitation.
DOI: https://doi.org/10.1016/B978-0-7020-8276-4.00004-7

With advances in acute medical and trauma care, rehabilitation teams are recognising an increasing number of patients surviving severe acquired brain injury but presenting in a prolonged disorder of consciousness (PDOC). The term PDOC encompasses the vegetative state (VS) and the minimally conscious state (MCS). It is inevitable that PDOC represents a clinically complex and ethically challenging scenario for rehabilitation teams and health care systems, and a life-changing situation for patients and their families.

*'I don't understand it. And before this happened to him, I never thought about it. I didn't even know that you could – you could be like that and still alive'.*
(*Mikaela, relative*, healthtalk.org)

In this area of practice, rehabilitation teams will be most successful if they take an interdisciplinary team (IDT) approach to assessment and treatment. By developing a thorough understanding of the range of PDOC presentations, rehabilitation teams will be equipped to diagnose these conditions and develop appropriate care and treatment plans. Teams should continuously consider available rehabilitation and treatment options within the context of the patient's best interests. By definition, such patients will not have capacity to make their own decisions so teams must ensure robust arrangements are in place to support decision making.

## Aims

1. To define PDOC and consider key differential diagnoses.
2. To describe assessment approaches as used in a pathway model of rehabilitation.
3. To understand challenges in providing PDOC assessment, care, and treatment.
4. To explore evolving and innovative practice in PDOC diagnosis.
5. To explore the evidence base for IDT working in PDOC.

## What is a prolonged disorder of consciousness?

A PDOC is a state which persists for more than 4 weeks following a sudden onset profound acquired brain injury (RCP, 2020). Patients in a PDOC will show no, or significantly reduced, signs of awareness to their surroundings. These patients have either limited or no functional method of communicating with the world. They appear suspended in a catastrophic new reality. With this in mind, you can begin to see the complexity of working with this patient cohort.

In VS there are no signs of awareness and no functional method of communication is observed. Where there are reproducible signs of awareness and attempts at communication, but they are minimal and/or inconsistent, this is known as a MCS. In both scenarios, the patient in a PDOC will lack the capacity to make decisions about their own care and situation, and will be unable to engage in conventional goal-orientated rehabilitation (RCP, 2020; Mental Capacity Act, 2005).

It can be challenging to reach an accurate diagnosis and to support families in understanding the PDOC condition. In VS it can be easy to inaccurately interpret reflexive movements and vocalisation as attempts at communication. In MCS the inconsistent presentation can be particularly difficult to assess. In addition to a complex assessment process, teams must balance the divergent views of individuals, clinicians, and the general public about the types of care and treatment that should be provided in severe brain injury. In order to manage these challenges a team-based approach is key.

The term 'low awareness state' is no longer desirable in current practice (PDOC has been adopted instead) as further detailed assessment may identify that a patient has no signs of awareness and no intention or ability to communicate (RCP, 2013). It is helpful to think about wakefulness (e.g., being awake or asleep) and awareness (e.g., being aware of self or environment) as separate entities, in order to understand the range of conditions covered by the PDOC spectrum (Table 4.1). In a coma state the patient is neither awake nor aware. In VS a person *can live and grow, but cannot sense or perceive'* (RCP, 2020). The patient has sleep–wake cycles unlike in coma. They will spend part of a 24-hour period with their eyes open although sleep–wake cycles may be severely disrupted. However, they do not show signs of awareness. In VS there are no signs of functional communication; however, it is important for rehabilitation teams to be aware of the range of reflexive and spontaneous responses which are compatible with this diagnosis.

Careful recording, assessment, and documentation are essential, as certain responses seen in VS can be misinterpreted as meaningful; for example, teeth grinding, spontaneous facial movements such as smiling or grimacing, spontaneous crying, and vocalisation such as grunting or groaning (all of which may be incorrectly interpreted as communicative attempts). Some responses, such as smiling, may be a basic reflex response, or in other instances may indicate a differentiating response that conveys emotional and communicative intent. Such a differentiating response would demonstrate more complex cognitive processing, for example, using smiling as a nonverbal method of making a choice. The grasp reflex, and purposeless movements of the limbs and/or trunk, may be observed in VS. It is also possible to observe fleeting fixation or following a moving object or loud sound, however in a VS presentation this is typically very poorly sustained (RCP, 2013).

In MCS the patient has sleep and wake cycles which may be abnormal. There are accompanying minimal and/or inconsistent signs of awareness to their

**TABLE 4.1** Wakefulness, awareness, and communication in PDOC conditions and key differential diagnoses.

| Diagnosis | Wakefulness | Awareness | Communication |
|---|---|---|---|
| Coma | Not awake | Not aware | No communication |
| VS | Sleep–wake cycles (may be severely disrupted/abnormal) | No behavioural signs of awareness | No functional communication. Reflexive behaviours such as vocalisation or smiling may be misinterpreted as meaningful and/or indicating purposeful communication |
| MCS | Sleep–wake cycles (may be severely disrupted/abnormal) | Minimal and/or inconsistent behavioural signs of awareness that are reproducible | Minimal and/or inconsistent attempts to communicate. In MCS + presentation may be able to inconsistently indicate 'yes'/'no' or make a simple choice. Wide spectrum of communicative abilities requiring specialist assessment |
| *Key differential diagnosis (not PDOC)* | | | |
| Locked-in state | Sleep–wake cycles (may be severely fatigued) | Fully aware of self and environment | Can communicate to a functional and high level with support of AAC (alternative and augmentative communication) aids and make decisions about care and treatment |

MCS, *minimally conscious state;* MCS +, *minimally conscious state plus;* PDOC, *prolonged disorder of consciousness;* VS, *vegetative state.*

surroundings. There may be minimal and/or inconsistent attempts to communicate in a functional way, for example, by following a spoken or written instruction or indicating 'yes' or 'no'. These signs must be reproducible or sustained in one or more (Box 4.1, from RCP, 2020).

Whilst the clinical features of a PDOC may be seen in the context of the advanced stages of a progressive neurological condition, for example, multiple sclerosis or dementia; the scope of the current national guidelines is limited to sudden onset traumatic and nontraumatic brain injury, for example, head injury, intracranial bleed, or infection. Teams will explore a specific PDOC diagnosis (e.g., VS or MCS); however, they must ensure that the patient's care pathway and best interest decisions are not determined by a diagnostic label in isolation.

The current direction of travel within PDOC clinical practice is a move away from focusing purely on the precise diagnostic label (e.g., VS or MCS). The diagnostic label is no longer the main factor in weighing up legal decisions about withdrawal of treatment (RCP, 2020). However, the diagnosis is still relevant in showing the trajectory of change and to inform discussions about prognosis for recovering awareness and/or function (RCP, 2020). Defining what the patient can and cannot do and experience also influences the best interests assessment. Is this a quality of life that would be acceptable to this patient? Does the trajectory of change influence the timings of the care and treatment decisions in hand? Robust assessments are also vital to highlight those patients who are in a locked-in state rather than a PDOC. In the locked-in state (Table 4.1), a patient has relatively intact cognition and communication in the context of profound motor disability. This is one of the most important differential diagnoses of PDOC and missing it could deprive a patient, with the ability to make their own decisions, from doing so. For example, a patient in locked-in state may be able to communicate to a highly complex level using a communication aid.

## Assessment approaches within a pathway model of rehabilitation

PDOC is a clinical diagnosis requiring thorough and detailed assessment undertaken by experienced practitioners. The RCP (2020) recommends evaluation by a multidisciplinary team of clinicians who are expert in the assessment of cognition, communication, and motor function in the context of PDOC. The team may consist of rehabilitation medical and nursing staff, physiotherapy, occupational therapy, speech and language therapy, dietetics and clinical psychology, with additional support from social work, mental health, and psychiatry teams as required. Rehabilitation coordination teams may be involved to ensure that the patient is receiving care in the most appropriate setting and enhance communication between teams and families.

Clinical teams in critical care and acute settings can find recognition of the PDOC state challenging. Frequently, patients who require ongoing support in a critical care unit are rarely ready for formal PDOC assessment due to ongoing medical instability. It can be challenging to carry out robust assessments in a critical care unit due to the overstimulating surroundings. Therefore, in clinical practice, assessments for PDOC often have a much later starting point in the patient journey than the 4-week point highlighted in the RCP (2020) guidelines.

Specialist neurorehabilitation teams should be involved for interim advice and review at an early stage postinjury (in the first few days and weeks), to support acute and critical care colleagues, form early relationships with patients' families, and begin planning for future care. Recognition and referral to a specialist rehabilitation team for PDOC assessment should occur from 4 weeks post sudden-onset brain injury, if there are inconsistent signs of awareness and/or no functional method of communication.

It is likely that the number of PDOC cases may be underreported in the United Kingdom (Wade, 2018). There are a number of factors which impact on this including staff training in PDOC, limited specialist rehabilitation services, and availability of outreach services. In clinical practice, teams may be challenged with the attitude that these patients do not have rehabilitation needs due to lack of responses and perceived inability to benefit from rehabilitation. However, provision of early specialist IDT intervention will provide the best possible opportunity for accurate assessment, comprehensive disability management, and appropriate best interest decision making.

In terms of time frames for assessment, a longer monitoring period is acceptable when evaluating patients for a permanent or chronic diagnosis when they have sustained a traumatic brain injury versus a nontraumatic injury. The national clinical guidelines (RCP, 2020) outline the recommended time points for formal assessment of awareness using the below standard clinical assessments:

1. Wessex Head Injury Matrix (WHIM) (Shiel et al., 2000).
2. Coma Recovery Scale-Revised (CRS-R) (Giacino et al., 2004).

3. Sensory Modality Assessment and Rehabilitation Technique (Gill-Thwaites and Munday, 1997).

It is recommended one or more tools are used for assessment. The CRS-R is most widely used internationally, and if only one tool is used, it is recommended that this tool is selected. The tools provide complementary information and specialist centres will typically offer the full range, selecting assessments based on the individual needs of the patient (RCP, 2020).

Turner-Stokes et al. (2015) evaluated the WHIM tool as a serial assessment method for the first 6 months post brain injury. They reported that the trajectory of change is an important predictor of outcome and suggested that teams should utilise cohort data to inform decision making around rehabilitation pathways. Patients who are showing a rapidly improving trajectory on WHIM assessment may be suitable for continuing evaluation in an inpatient rehabilitation setting. In contrast, a patient with inconsistent scores and a flatter trajectory on the WHIM may benefit from a longer period of IDT evaluation, which may be provided outside of acute settings, for example, by slow stream rehabilitation centres or specialist community outreach teams experienced in PDOC management.

In practice, inpatient IDTs will need to meet regularly (at least weekly) to discuss suitable rehabilitation pathways for each patient given their specific needs and readiness for formal assessment. Teams should supplement weekly discussion with information gleaned from formal assessment tools and informal observations. IDTs will need to regularly consider best interests decision making within the relevant national legal frameworks.

At a service design level, it is imperative for commissioners to appreciate realistic time scales involved. The process of transferring a severely brain injured patient from a critical care environment to rehabilitation, optimising their disability management, and carrying out at least one thorough formal awareness assessment, can be lengthy (6 months+). Traditional rehabilitation outcome measures may not be sensitive to the PDOC caseload, for example, a Functional Impairment Measure and Functional Attainment Measure (FIM FAM) (Turner-Stokes et al., 1999) score may be the same on admission and discharge despite a comprehensive assessment and management programme being delivered.

The national clinical guidelines describe a revolving door policy, to ensure that patients who have been discharged from hospital to slower stream rehabilitation or specialist care facilities, are able to reaccess more intensive specialist rehabilitation services if they show signs of change. It is helpful to agree on patient-specific targets that describe behaviours in a clear way so that families and carers can recognise and report meaningful changes. Referrals back into services should be screened by a rehabilitation practitioner with appropriate experience in PDOC.

Clinical rehabilitation teams will need to regularly assess using formal and informal structured measures. Assessment choice, approach, and timing will be influenced by multiple factors (Fig. 4.1). IDT involvement is essential in

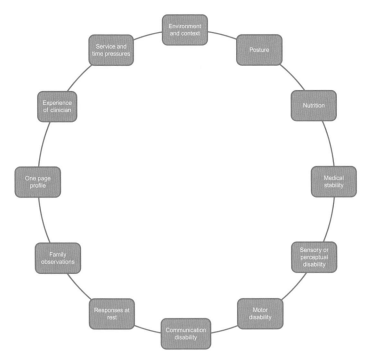

FIGURE 4.1   Factors to be considered when undertaking PDOC assessment. From Royal College of Physicians. Prolonged disorders of consciousness following sudden onset brain injury: National clinical guidelines. London: RCP, 2020. Copyright © 2020 Royal College of Physicians. Reproduced with permission.

diagnosis as specific professions are experts in some of the features that commonly disguise awareness. For example, a speech and language therapist (SLT) can guide in the differential diagnosis between global aphasia and PDOC and crucially in patients who may be locked in. The physiotherapist and occupational therapist can evaluate movements towards an object, such as a feedback switch (e.g., buzzer) to establish if the movement is reproducible and purposeful or if it is a movement seen at rest or as part of a generalised tonal pattern. These examples highlight that assessment should not depend upon isolated individuals whatever their profession and expertise individually (RCP, 2013).

IDTs should strive to find out about the patient's life and family experiences prior to their brain injury as part of person-centred care. Completing a *One-Page Profile* (Poulter, 2016) can be a useful technique in engaging families in this work. Teams should ensure that they see the individual (and their personality) and not just the patient (and their medical condition), by considering what motivates the patient and what is important to them.

Where the patient has no intentional communication or inconsistent communication, teams will rely on families to fill in the gaps. Latchem et al. (2015)

highlight that person-centred care is crucial in the context of PDOC, where the patient risks being treated as 'just a body'. Families typically spend more time with their loved one than individual clinicians or IDTs, therefore observations made by family members form an important part of assessment. Patients may be more likely to respond to a familiar person, therefore involving loved ones in sessions can help clinicians to observe responses and to provide education about their loved one's condition. Clinical psychologists may provide specifically tailored support to families of patients receiving PDOC assessment and rehabilitation.

The assessment setting may inhibit or enhance all types of response and behaviours, and therefore must be given full consideration. A quiet environment, such as a side room or treatment room, is essential for carrying out formal assessment such as the WHIM, CRS-R, or Sensory Modality Assessment and Rehabilitation Technique assessment. Clinical teams may also utilise informal tools such as the Putney PDOC Toolkit (Wilford et al., 2018). It is good practice to compare the responses of the patient when at rest with no external stimulation, to their responses when presented with a range of stimuli covering all sensory modalities (e.g., visual, auditory, tactile, olfactory, and gustatory). Sensory assessment techniques should be adequately risk assessed, for example, sense of smell will be impacted by the presence of a cuffed tracheostomy tube and using tastes should be risk assessed considering dysphagia assessment findings. Carrying out assessments with staff from different professions within the IDT can help to reach consensus on responses. It may be helpful to film behaviours and consider responses as a whole team (Pundole et al., 2019).

Optimisation of the patient's condition, environment, and using a consistent team approach to assessment involving loved ones, is more important than the choice of assessment tool. Teams should consider and document responses in any situation. Nursing staff play a significant role here as they observe the patient outside of formal therapy sessions. In this way, teams can provide a 24-hour assessment. For example, during a routine activity such as toothbrushing a range of responses could be seen:

- no response to task or objects;
- reflexive responses such as startle when the brush is put into the mouth or clamping down of teeth to the brush;
- withdrawal type responses whereby the patient pulls away or closes their eyes;
- localising responses whereby the patient follows objects with their eyes and reaches out towards the toothbrush;
- discriminating responses whereby the patient shows ability to use the objects (toothbrush or toothpaste) functionally, follows basic instructions or uses facial expression to express like or dislike to the flavour of the toothpaste versus the flavour of a lip balm;

- responses indicating emergence such as consistently using objects, following instructions or making communicative attempts in the context of this everyday task.

Carrying out informal sessions in a range of contexts, such as a café or garden (Pundole et al., 2019) may be more stimulating for the patient and therefore more likely to elicit a response. Assessment should take place at different times of the day, to evaluate any patterns that may optimise responses. Such sessions complement formal assessments and provide opportunities for responses within a person-centred context. Taking a patient into a garden may provide opportunity to observe response to a variety of scents. Facilitating a visit from a family pet may provide a motivating context to observe responses such as tracking, purposeful use of objects (e.g., treat, lead, and brush), and communicative attempts.

Consideration of posture and positioning will impact on the quality of assessment. Being in an upright supported posture is likely to have a positive impact on ability to remain wakeful and to respond. Teams will explore the impact of position on responses by comparing results when in different positions, for example, seated in a wheelchair versus on a tilt table. Latchem et al. (2015) describe how professionals' and families' perceptions of the aims of physiotherapy input can differ and that communication is crucial to reducing the distress to families. They describe how families' perceptions of interventions (e.g., tilt table or tracheostomy care) may change over time; therefore, it is important to have regular family meetings to explore the clinical rationale for interventions and to explain what is involved (e.g., what families can expect to see and hear within a session).

Ensuring medical stability prior to formal assessment is crucial. Seizures, hydrocephalus, electrolyte/hormonal imbalance, infection, and pain could all affect a patient's responses during assessment (see Chapter 2) and must be addressed. Review of medications which may affect awareness prior to assessment is essential. Any changes to medication during assessment periods should be noted, including any subsequent impact on assessment scores. In some cases, specific medications are trialled to enhance awareness; medical teams will take the lead on this and should discuss treatment carefully with the IDT before and throughout a trial. Clinicians carrying out PDOC assessment should alert medical staff to changes in the responses seen as these may highlight a medical deterioration which can be subtle in a patient with PDOC. Dhamapurkar et al. (2018) describe the use of serial WHIM assessment not only to monitor cognitive change over time but also to highlight underlying physical change such as infection. A dietitian will advise on optimal timings of assessments, particularly the use of formal tools which are best started when a patient is nutritionally stable. Montalcini et al. (2015) identified that MCS patients with lower serum albumin had significantly higher short-term mortality than those with higher serum albumin. Comprehensive dietetic assessment is therefore an essential prerequisite to commencing assessments for PDOC.

## Challenges in providing assessment, care, and treatment for PDOC

Physical, sensory, and communication impairments are major factors that can mask signs of awareness. Multimodal assessment techniques are therefore recommended due to the likelihood of concomitant disability in the severely brain injured patient. Andrews et al. (1996) carried out a retrospective review of patients admitted to a specialist rehabilitation unit with a diagnosis of VS. They showed that the misdiagnosis rate was 43%, with 17 of the 40 patients included in the study had been wrongly presumed to be in VS. Crucially, most of the wrongly diagnosed patients had a visual impairment and all were severely physically disabled. The authors found that 15 out of 17 patients were able to communicate their preference in some quality-of-life issues, and six were rated as orientated, purposeful, and appropriate on the Racho scale (Whyte, 2011).

Martin Pistorious (Pistorius, 2015), who suffered a severe brain injury due to an infection in childhood, powerfully describes, from a patient perspective, the experience of signs of awareness being missed and of awareness returning. This is an atypical and extreme case and this level of recovery will not be borne out in the vast majority. However, it must serve to remind clinicians that when we think we have found the answer, we should keep looking.

> *'Meanwhile, my mind began knitting itself back together. Gradually, my awareness started to return. But no one realized that I had come back to life. I was aware of everything, just like any normal person. I could see and understand everything, but I couldn't find a way to let anybody know. My personality was entombed within a seemingly silent body, a vibrant mind hidden in plain sight within a chrysalis'.*
>
> *(Pistorius, 2015)*

The rates of misdiagnosis in PDOC highlight the need for a gold standard IDT approach. The higher-level responses that indicate emergence from MCS (e.g., functional object use, command following, and expressive communication) are not easily interpreted by clinicians working in isolation. For example, an occupational therapist assessing object use during personal care may need to work alongside a physiotherapist to understand the achievable movement patterns, tone issues, coordination, and optimal positioning of that patient for that task. The team should have an understanding of the movements seen at rest, in order to assess if responses are in relation to the stimuli used. Does the response occur without stimulation or can it be assigned to a specific stimuli-related response? If emergence from MCS is signalled by object use, an occupational therapist could work with the patient to facilitate and evaluate the consistency of functional object use in everyday activity.

SLTs have a key role in the assessment, management, and monitoring of patients in PDOC due to the emphasis on communication behaviours in the definitions used to determine MCS and emergence (Pundole et al., 2019). The SLT will work with the team to discuss the level of language complexity and psycholinguistic components of instructions given to the patient. The SLT will advise on factors that influence the anticipated type of expressive communication, for example, severe orofacial weakness increases the likelihood of a dysarthria. Therefore planning to assess with alternative simple augmentative and alternative communication methods such as a communication chart may be helpful. Instructions should be given verbally and in written format due to potential auditory or visual disturbances. Response reliability and consistency should be probed using a range of resources and contexts.

The medical team will need to consider, with specialist input from the IDT, the introduction and management of clinically assisted nutrition and hydration (CANH). The disorders of consciousness have been described as the unintended consequence of advances in early management of neurological damage (Laureys et al., 2006; Healy, 2010). Clinicians and families who find themselves caring for a patient in a PDOC will need to engage with a range of ethical questions as time passes, and the PDOC may become a chronic condition. One of the foremost issues in clinical practice, and in research in recent times, has been the withdrawal of medical treatments that may be life-sustaining, including CANH. Teams and families caring for patients in a PDOC are required to ensure that the provision and continuation of medical treatments including CANH are within the patient's best interests. In terms of weighing up best interests for any treatment, it is important to consider:

- any formal documented evidence that the patient had prior to the brain injury (such as an 'Advance Decision to Refuse Treatment');
- a holistic view of the patient's likely views and opinions if they were able to contribute (which may include information from relatives, friends, and colleagues);
- a strong ethical presumption in favour of sustaining life;
- the current status of the patient in terms of their medical needs and PDOC diagnosis;
- the trajectory of change over time;
- the likely 'best case' and 'worst case' scenarios; is this an outcome or quality of life that would be acceptable to the patient if they were able to express a view?

Clinicians must ensure that assessments are robust, detailed, and carried out by appropriately experienced staff. In the United Kingdom, there are national guidelines that support teams in this area, such as RCP (2020) and BMA (2018). Consultation with legal support services may be required. In the United Kingdom/England, withdrawal of CANH in PDOC is no longer automatically referred to the Court of Protection if all parties are in agreement with a best interests decision; robust processes within the current legal framework and safeguards such as expert second clinical opinions are in place.

## Evolving and innovative practice in PDOC diagnosis

Current diagnoses within the PDOC spectrum are based on the behavioural signs of awareness observed by specialist teams. Research studies employing neuroimaging, for example, functional magnetic resonance imaging (fMRI), which shows blood flow to areas of cortical activity, have been used with PDOC patients. Studies have demonstrated islands of cortical functioning in patients who were clinically diagnosed with VS (Healy, 2010). Owen et al. (2006) showed that when asked to imagine playing tennis, cortical areas were activated so that an fMRI scan of a patient diagnosed with VS was matched to a healthy control. Whilst these technologies are not currently utilised in clinical practice, teams should be aware that our current understanding of consciousness is limited, and clinical observations are reflections—rather than direct measurements—of cortical activity.

Wang et al. (2019) studied responses to verbal instructions to elicit a basic motor movement (hand raising) in 29 patients in a PDOC using fMRI and matched healthy controls. They found activity of the motor-related cortical network, which was not elicited during standard behavioural assessment, for four patients. Three of these patients who demonstrated changes on fMRI scan showed improvements with their CRS-R scores at 3, 6, and 12 months, whilst 9 out of 25 remaining patients showed improvement on longitudinal clinical assessment. Within this limited sample size, it is not yet possible to ascertain the relevance of such fMRI changes in PDOC. However, Wang et al. (2019) assert that clinicians should consider the capacity for covert cognitive processing beyond overt signs of awareness when conducting diagnostic behavioural assessment. Bender et al. (2015) describe the potential for a category of patients in a 'subclinical MCS'.

The findings from fMRI studies challenge our understanding of consciousness and how to assess it. However, Lugo et al. (2019) report a lack of effectiveness in practical applications of technology, stating that whilst academically thought provoking, they are not yet utilised clinically. Whilst the diagnostic categories of VS and MCS were given significant weight in previous clinical guidelines (RCP, 2013), and remain the focus of the main assessment tools, teams must not neglect continual assessment of the patient's best interests. Diagnosis must not determine decisions about care and treatment. Discovering that a particular movement can light up an area of motor cortex on an fMRI scan may challenge a diagnosis, however, may not always contradict a best interest decision. Scan findings, such as those shown in the Owen et al. (2006) study, are unlikely to be functionally useful or alter the patient's quality of life.

Soeterik (2017) reports that the type of diagnosis within the PDOC spectrum does not influence the family's experience of distress. Willmot and White (2017) question whether it is even clinically useful or legally necessary to define patients as VS or MCS. Teams must keep up-to-date with technological advances however continue to balance diagnostic information from standard clinical assessment or from innovative technologies, with the best interests of that patient and their family.

## Developing effective and evidence-based team working for PDOC

When working with a patient in a PDOC, it is imperative to work across traditional professional boundaries in order to assess the patient's level of awareness and attempt to establish functional communication methods; an IDT approach here is essential. Clinicians who are inexperienced in working with PDOC require support, particularly in relation to extended practice roles. It is acknowledged that there is a general lack of exposure to PDOC in preregistration training (Logeswaren et al., 2018). Even for experienced clinicians, it can be a challenge to apply generic skills to an unfamiliar and complex patient group.

When a patient is seemingly not responding at all, it can be difficult to know where to start. There is a growing body of research, continuing professional development (CPD), and education resources to guide professionals in this area (Munday, 2005; Roberts and Greenwood, 2019). There is an increasing range of profession specific guidelines (e.g., Pundole et al., 2019; RCP Guidelines, 2020) to underpin the knowledge and skills required to work with this challenging condition.

Logeswaren et al. (2018) explored the views of staff working with patients with a PDOC in a specialist rehabilitation unit. They found that medical, nursing, and allied health professionals identified five key themes related to the positive aspects of working with the PDOC caseload. These were: seeing change, supporting families, providing a quality team-based clinical input, the complexity of the work, and the personal impact of the work. Negative themes identified were: dealing with death and 'living death' scenarios, dealing with family expectations and distress, and the negative impact on staff on both professional and personal levels. Soeterik (2017) identifies that in order to support families well, you also need to support the professionals who work with them. However, families and professionals may have fundamentally different expectations around recovery, deviating goals, and contradictory feelings which can be a source of conflict (Span Sluyter et al., 2018). The aims of specialist rehabilitation services are commonly centred around assessment, disability management, and discharge. These aims may not be aligned with families' goals around active rehabilitation and hope of recovery.

Soeterik (2017) describes how these divergent views of the rehabilitation pathway and disagreements about assessment findings can lead to feelings of abandonment and conflict by families, for example, as interventions are withdrawn. Soeterik highlights the work of Jox et al. (2015) that found 24% of families disagreed with formal assessment results and maintained high hope that the person in PDOC would be able to communicate in the future. The shift away from emphasis on diagnostic labels towards considering the best interests of the individual may be helpful to IDTs in managing these divergent expectations.

Understanding that the IDTs' aims and objectives during the rehabilitation pathway may differ from the families' expectations is essential. Soeterik (2017) reports that families may find interactions with health care professionals distressing, and that health care professionals have also reported interactions with family members to be distressing to them leading to burn out. Clinicians working within the PDOC field should ensure that there are frequent opportunities for open and transparent communication with families and appropriate clinical supervision and support.

## Summary

Specialist rehabilitation teams are being referred increasing numbers of patients who may be in a PDOC. Assessing and managing these patients require specialist skills, clinical support, and an appropriate environment. Working within an IDT framework is essential in order to reach a valid diagnosis. Current understanding of human consciousness is being challenged by technological advances, therefore rehabilitation teams will increasingly need to balance scientific developments with family expectations and capacity of health care services. However, teams must also consider PDOC diagnoses within the wider context of the best interests of the individual patient. To provide an effective rehabilitation pathway following the most severe of brain injuries, an IDT approach, including health care professionals and family members, is vital, with the patient at the centre.

**Reflective questions**

Consider a severely brain injured patient you have worked with. What type of behavioural responses did you observe and what might indicate about their level of awareness?

How would you explain a rehabilitation pathway for PDOC to a patient's loved ones? How would you ensure that your assessment and treatment processes were holistic, robust, and in the individual's best interests?

Thinking about what your own wishes would be in the event of a severe brain injury can be a useful starting point to understanding your own opinions about quality of life and best interests. Discuss this with your family, friends, colleagues, or student peers and consider the range of views that are relevant to the PDOC caseload.

Consider your professional role when working with this patient group. How might your working practices, IDT working, professional development, and clinical supervision needs be changed when working in this context?

# References

Andrews, K., Murphy, L., Munday, R., Littlewood, C., 1996. Misdiagnosis of the vegetative state: retrospective study in a rehabilitation unit. BMJ 313, 13.

Bender, A., Jox, R., Grill, E., Straube, A., Lulé, D., 2015. Persistent vegetative state and minimally conscious state. A systematic review and meta-analysis of diagnostic procedures. Dtsch Arztebl Int 112 (14): 235–242.

British Medical Association (BMA). 2018. Clinically-assisted nutrition and hydration (CANH). New guidance to support doctors making decisions about CANH for adults who lack capacity in England and Wales. Available at: https://www.bma.org.uk/advice/employment/ethics/mental-ecapacity/clinically-assisted-nutrition-and-hydration. Accessed January 22, 2020.

Dhamapurkar, S.K., Wilson, B.A., Rose, A., Florschutz, G., Watson, P., Shiel, A., 2018. Does a regular Wessex Head Injury Matrix assessment identify early signs of infections in people with prolonged disorders of consciousness? Brain Injury 32 (9), 1103–1109.

Giacino, J.T., Kalmar, K., Whyte, J., 2004. The JFK coma recovery scale-revised: measurement characteristics and diagnostic utility. Arch. Phys. Med. Rehab. 85, 2020–2029.

Gill-Thwaites, H., 1997. The Sensory Modality Assessment Rehabilitation Technique – a tool for assessment and treatment of patients with severe brain injury in a vegetative state. Brain Injury 11, 723–734.

Healy, J., 2010. The vegetative state: life, death and consciousness. J. Intensive Care Soc. 11 (2), 118–123. Available at: http://www.healthtalk.org/peoples-experiences/nerves-brain/family-exp eriences-vegetative-and-minimally-conscious-states/messages-healthcare-professionals-service -providers-policy-makers. Accessed October 27, 2019.

Jox, R.J., Kuehlmeyer, K., Klein, A.M., Herzog, J., Schaupp, M., Nowak, D.A., Koenig, E., Müller, F., Bender, A., 2015. Diagnosis and decision making for patients with disorders of consciousness: a survey among family members. Arch. Phys. Med. Rehabil. 96 (2), 323–330.

Latchem, J., Kitzinger, J., Kitzinger, C., 2015. Physiotherapy for vegetative and minimally conscious state patients: family perceptions and experiences. Disabil. Rehab. 38 (1), 22–29.

Laureys, S., Boly, M., Maquet, P., 2006. Tracking the recovery of consciousness from coma. J. Clin. Invest. 116, 1823–1825.

Logeswaran, S., Papps, B., Turner-Stokes, L., 2018. Staff experiences of working with patients with prolonged disorders of consciousness: a focus group analysis. Int. J. Therapy Rehab. 25 (11), 602–612.

Lugo Z., Pokorny C., Pellas F., Noirhomme Q., Laureys S., Müller-Putz G. and Kübler A. 2019. Mental imagery for brain–computer interface control and communication in non-responsive individuals. Ann. Phys. Rehab. Med. 63 (1), 21–27. 10.1016/j.rehab.2019.02.005.

Mental Capacity Act. 2005. Available at: https://www.legislation.gov.uk/ukpga/2005/9/contents. Accessed October 28, 2019.

Montalcini, T., Moraca, M., Ferro, Y., Romeo, S., Serra, S., Raso, M.G., Pujia, A., 2015. Nutritional parameters predicting pressure ulcers and short-term mortality in patients with minimal conscious state as a result of traumatic and non-traumatic acquired brain injury. J. Transl. Med. 13, 305.

Munday, R., 2005. Vegetative and minimally conscious states: how can occupational therapists help? Neuropsychol. Rehab. 15 (3–4), 503–513.

Owen, A.M., Coleman, M.R., Boly, M., Davis, M.H., Laureys, S., Pickard, J.D., 2006. Detecting awareness in the vegetative state. Science 8 (5792), 1402 313.

Pistorious M. 2015. How my mind came back to life – and no one knew. TED talk. Available at: https://www.ted.com/talks/martin_pistorius_how_my_mind_came_back_to_life_and_no_one_ knew. Accessed October 28, 2019.

Poulter, GP-123, 2016. Using one page profiles to improve person centred care on the inpatient unit (IPU). BMJ Support. Palliat. Care 6, A54–A55.

Pundole, A., Ankers, M., Clarkson, K., Harp, K., Mills, C., Roberts, H., 2019. Guidelines for Speech and Language Therapists Working With Adults in a Disorder of Consciousness. Developed by a UK Wide Group of Speech and Language Therapists. Royal Hospital for Neurodisability, London.

Roberts, H., Greenwood, N., 2019. Speech and language therapy best practice for patients in prolonged disorders of consciousness: a modified Delphi study. Int. J. Lang. Commun. Disord. 54 (5), 841–854.

Royal College of Physicians. 2013. Prolonged Disorders of Consciousness: National Clinical Guidelines (Report of a Working Party). Royal College of Physicians, London.

Royal College of Physicians, 2020. Prolonged Disorders of Consciousness Following Sudden Onset Brain Injury. National Clinical Guidelines. Royal College of Physicians, London.

Shiel, A., Horn, S.A., Wilson, B.A., Elder, V., McCrudden, E., 2000. The Wessex Head Injury Matrix – Manual. Pearson Assessment, London.

Soeterik, S., 2017. The Experience of Families and Healthcare Professionals Supporting People With Prolonged Disorders of Consciousness. Royal Holloway, University of London.

Span-Sluyter, C., Lavrijsen, J., van Leeuwen, E., 2018. Moral dilemmas and conflicts concerning patients in a vegetative state/unresponsive wakefulness syndrome: shared or non-shared decision making? A qualitative study of the professional perspective in two moral case deliberations. BMC Med. Ethics 19, 10.

Turner-Stokes, L., Bassett, P., Rose, H., Ashford, S., Thu, A., 2015. Serial measurement of Wessex Head Injury Matrix in the diagnosis of patients in vegetative and minimally conscious states: a cohort analysis. BMJ Open 5, e006051. doi:10.1136/bmjopen-2014-006051.

Turner-Stokes, L., Nyein, K., Turner-Stokes, T., Gatehouse, C., 1999. The UK FIM+FAM: development and evaluation. Functional assessment measure. Clin. Rehab. 13 (4), 277–287.

Wade, D., 2018. How many patients in a prolonged disorder of consciousness might need a best interests meeting about starting or continuing gastrostomy feeding? Clin. Rehab. 32 (11), 1551–1564.

Wang, F., Hu, N., Hu, X., Jing, S., Heine, L., Thibaut, A., Huang, W., Yan, Y., Wang, J., Schnakers, C., Laureys, S., Di, H., 2019. Detecting brain activity following a verbal command in patients with disorders of consciousness. Front. Neurosci. 13, 976.

Whyte, J., 2011. Rancho Los Amigos Scale. In: Kreutzer, J.S., DeLuca, J., Caplan, B. (Eds.), Encyclopedia of Clinical Neuropsychology. Springer, New York, NY.

Wilford S., Pundole A., Crawford S., Hanrahan A. 2018. The Putney PDOC Toolkit. Available at: https://www.rhn.org.uk/research/putney-prolonged-disorder-of-consciousness-toolkit/. Accessed September 26, 2021.

Willmott, L., White, B., 2017. Persistent vegetative state and minimally conscious state: ethical, legal and practical dilemas. J. Med. Ethics 43, 425–426.

## Chapter 5

# 24-hour approach to physical management

Emily Wilson-Meredith and Emily Low

## Chapter outline

### Abstract

*Objective*: To describe the physical problems encountered by patients after complex injury/illness; explain the rationale behind a 24-hour approach to the physical management of patients; highlight the benefits of good physical management and the risks of poor management; and to describe a range of interdisciplinary treatment modalities used to optimise the physical status of patients within rehabilitation.

*Background*: Rehabilitation is a 24-hour process involving all members of the interdisciplinary team, the patient, and their family/carers. Physical and postural management may be required throughout the patients' rehabilitation journey, and for those with

A Practical Approach to Interdisciplinary Complex Rehabilitation.
DOI: https://doi.org/10.1016/B978-0-7020-8276-4.00005-9

residual physical impairment, it may continue long after all rehabilitation goals are met, for maintenance, and to prevent future complications.

*Main concepts explored*: Physical consequences of complex illness/injury (muscle weakness, altered muscle tone, spatial neglect, apraxia, ataxia and other movement disorders, contractures, fractures, amputation, altered blood pressure, vestibular problems, and respiratory compromise); the role of the interdisciplinary team in physical management, treatment modalities (positioning, seating, stretching, orthoses, taping/strapping/support garments, electrical stimulation, constraint-induced movement therapy, mechanical adjuncts, surgical and medical management, environmental adjustments, and assistive technology) and discharge planning.

**Keywords**
Physical management; Rehabilitation; 24-hour; Interdisciplinary team; Physiotherapy; Occupational therapy

## Aims

1. To describe the physical issues encountered by patients after complex injury/illness.
2. To explain the rationale behind a 24-hour approach to the physical management of patients undergoing rehabilitation.
3. To highlight the benefits of good physical management and the risks of poor management.
4. To describe a selection of the interdisciplinary treatment modalities used to optimise the physical status of patients within rehabilitation.

## Introduction

Rehabilitation is a 24-hour process involving all members of the interdisciplinary team (IDT), the patient, and their family/carers. A physical rehabilitation programme consists of structured therapy sessions, self-directed exercise, and postural management, as well as providing opportunity for rest. The optimisation of a person's physical status is important as it can improve engagement in all aspects of their rehabilitation, promote gains in function and independence, and reduce the risk of complications associated with periods of immobility. Physical and postural management may be required throughout the patients' rehabilitation journey and, for those with residual physical impairment, could continue as maintenance long after all rehabilitation goals are met, to prevent future complications.

This chapter will describe the physical issues commonly encountered during complex rehabilitation, along with some of the interventions an IDT may use to support physical optimisation. The interventions are appropriate for a range of diagnoses and functional levels, and are supported by both clinical experience and the research literature.

## Physical consequences of injury/illness

Patients admitted to a complex rehabilitation setting may have physical impairments and require careful consideration of their environment, treatment, positioning, and handling. Impairments may be a result of trauma, new or long-standing neurological or musculoskeletal conditions, comorbidities (such as arthritis, COPD, and spina bifida), or may have developed following a prolonged inpatient stay. Below we will discuss some of the problems commonly affecting this patient group.

### Muscle wasting

Muscle wasting can occur in certain neurological and musculoskeletal conditions, and in situations where the muscles have not been active for prolonged periods of time. Where wasting is a result of a progressive neurological condition or severe damage to the nerve or muscle, improvement may not be seen despite physical intervention. Where the underlying muscles and nerves are healthy, the prognosis is typically good.

Immobility and bed rest can be detrimental to patients. An average of 20–30% muscle wastage can occur in patients who remain in bed for over 1 week (Parry, 2015). Physiological changes in the muscle tissue include absorption of sarcomeres, increase in fatty and connective tissue, and the formation of adhesions within the joint capsule. Other consequences include respiratory muscle wastage (increasing susceptibility to chest infections), decreased bone density (increasing risk of fractures), joint stiffness and/or loss of range of motion, and reduced exercise tolerance. The treatment of muscle wasting may include stretches, strengthening, body weight supported exercises, and early mobilisation.

### Muscle weakness

Weakness refers to loss of muscle strength. Many people with normal muscle strength say they feel weak when the problem is actually fatigue, or when their movement is limited because of pain or joint stiffness. Muscle weakness can be a symptom of nervous system malfunction, physical damage to the muscle tissue, prolonged use of certain drugs, immobility, and/or a disease process.

Physiotherapy and occupational therapy can help people maintain, and sometimes regain, strength, or support them as they adapt to permanent weakness and compensate for loss of function.

### Altered muscle tone

Muscle tone has been described in a multitude of ways, however neither a precise definition nor a quantitative measure has been determined. In simple terms, tone is related to the levels of contractility and relaxation of muscle. It is typically discussed in terms of hypertonia (increased tone), hypotonia (reduced tone), or dystonia (variable tone). Altered muscle tone is seen within neurological illness or injury, and the type of tonal problem depends on whether the upper motor neurons (nerves within the brain or spinal cord) or the lower motor neurons (peripheral nerves that have exited the spine and travel through the body to muscles) are damaged. Following an upper motor neuron injury, muscle signs can be classified as positive (an *increased* response) or negative (a *decreased* response). Positive responses include: hypertonia or spasticity, rigidity, exaggerated reflexes, clonus, and associated reactions. Negative responses include muscle weakness and hypotonia. Lower motor neuron injuries are distinct from upper motor neuron injuries in that they present with mostly negative signs including: muscle wasting, fasciculations (muscle twitching), decreased reflexes, hypotonia, and weakness.

## Hypotonia

Following a brain or spinal injury, tone in affected muscles will start off low. If the injury is severe, there is often a period of flaccidity (total relaxation of the muscle). This will vary in duration, and some patients may be left with long-standing hypotonia, whilst others may gradually develop hypertonia or spasticity.

Patients with injuries to the peripheral nerves will also present with reduced tone which may improve over time with rehabilitation, but unfortunately, this can also be persistent for some patients.

With hypotonia, joints become vulnerable as the ligaments within them are able to stretch and the surrounding musculature is no longer able to support the joint position. This means that joints can become unstable and even partially dislocate (sublux) or completely dislocate. This is seen commonly in the shoulder joint following stroke. Careful positioning and use orthoses are key in the management of hypotonia.

## Spasticity

Spasticity has been described as 'disordered sensorimotor control, resulting from an upper motor neuron lesion, presenting as an intermittent or sustained involuntary activation of muscles' (Pandyan et al., 2005).

Spasticity can result from injury to the brain or spinal cord. It mainly affects the 'antigravity' muscles of the arm (flexors) and leg (extensors). Spasticity has been shown to develop and peak at 1–3 months postinjury (Wissel et al., 2013). The muscular components of spasticity may continue to progress beyond this time period, and such progression may lead to contractures (despite good management in many cases).

Spasticity does not merit treatment unless it is causing significant impairment and/or complications. For some, spasticity can be beneficial as it can aid with postural support and help keep the patient upright when their muscles are weak. In such cases, spasticity can facilitate standing/walking and subsequently support the preservation of bone density and muscle mass. For some patients, however, spasticity can cause issues with pain, positioning, movement, and hygiene. Physical treatment including positioning, splinting, and stretching is the mainstay, but medical adjuncts may be required to effectively manage spasticity.

## Rigidity

In contrast to spasticity there is no period of 'free movement', and rigidity is not velocity dependent. The muscles of an affected limb stiffen and resist passive movement. Rigidity involves both flexor and extensor groups, however, is more prominent in muscles that maintain a flexed posture. It may be accompanied by 'cogwheel' phenomenon (especially in patients with Parkinsonism) where the muscles intermittently catch and release during the movement. A stretching programme may be helpful where rigidity is a problem.

## Clonus

Clonus can develop after brain or spinal injury and is seen as rhythmic, involuntary muscle contractions. The first contraction (known as a clonic beat) is the longest, and decreases in length with each beat. It may be seen at the ankle (most commonly), patella, triceps, jaw, wrist, and biceps. It is often precipitated by sudden movement. Pain and cold are the leading cutaneous stimuli giving rise to, and sustaining, clonus (Boyraz et al., 2015). It is thought to be caused by a self-re-excitation of hyperactive stretch reflexes (Hilder and Rymer, 1999). Clonus is not usually painful but can interfere with posture and activity. Management may include stretching, orthoses, and medical interventions.

## Dystonia

Dystonia is a movement disorder where patients experience sustained or intermittent muscle contractions causing abnormal, often repetitive, movements, postures, or both. Dystonic movements are typically patterned, twisting, and may involve a tremor. Like spasticity and clonus, it may respond to physical and medical management.

## Associated reactions

These are abnormal reflex activities which may occur in the absence of voluntary movements. The incidence is poorly known. Commonly seen reactions are upper limb flexion and lower limb extension on yawning, or upper limb flexion when walking.

Associated reactions can affect balance and may be aesthetically frustrating for patients. They can be challenging to manage; modalities may include stretching, orthoses, and medical management.

## Spatial neglect

Spatial neglect is seen when a patient is not fully aware of the external space on one side of their body, or aware of that side of their body at all. It occurs in up to 50% of right hemispheric stroke survivors (Li, 2015). Patients with spatial neglect may not notice items on the affected side, meaning they may not be able to feed themselves, make a drink, or use a call bell to gain help. They may also be at risk of 'forgetting' affected limbs which may get trapped or left in a poor position. Another complication that can arise, secondary to spatial neglect, is that the person rests with their neck rotated to one side which causes muscle shortening, pain, and decreased range of movement. They may struggle to return their gaze to midline, creating a vicious cycle, with further decreased awareness of the neglected side and a decreased ability to move to that side. Encouraging a patient to scan to their affected side during tasks can be helpful.

## Apraxia

Apraxia (also referred to as dyspraxia) is an acquired disorder of motor planning, caused by damage to specific areas of the brain (most often left sided, involving the frontal and parietal lobes). Patients may be able to perform involuntary actions, but cannot repeat them voluntarily, or they may perseverate on certain movements. There are many different types of apraxia which can affect the movements of the face, limbs, and eyes. People with apraxia/dyspraxia need to work on retraining movements and relearning sequencing in order to increase functional independence. Apraxia is further considered in Chapter 9.

## Ataxia

Ataxia causes loss of fluid muscle movements, proprioception (awareness of position of the body), balance, and coordination. Most types of ataxia are caused by cerebellar lesions and muscle power is not normally affected. Some people inherit conditions causing ataxia via specific genes that have come from one or both parents. Some develop ataxia due to vitamin deficiencies, degeneration of the balance center, or prolonged exposure to high levels of alcohol. Others can develop ataxia from a stroke, tumour, viral infection, or head injury (Ataxia UK, 2014). Options for the treatment of ataxia include dynamic task practice (challenges stability and explores stability limits), strength and flexibility training, compensatory approaches (e.g., orthotics, movement retraining, and optimising the environment), weighted cuffs, and cooling (to reduce tremor).

## Other movement disorders

Other disorders include (but are not limited to) hemiballismus (an uncontrollable, poorly patterned flinging movement of an entire limb, which follows an infarction of the subthalamic nucleus), athetosis (characterised by the inability to sustain the fingers, toes, tongue, or any other body part in one position, as it is interrupted by slow, sinuous, purposeless movements), and chorea (involuntary arrhythmic movements of a forcible, jerky, and rapid nature). People who demonstrate these kinds of movement are at risk of further injury due to shearing or the blunt force of the moving limbs against their surroundings. These disorders can be challenging to manage and may require medical intervention. Equipment and handling advice to support patient and carer safety can be provided by the IDT.

## Contractures

Contractures can form in patients with or without a neurological injury. The sequence of formation of contractures is unclear, however anyone with a limb held with its muscles in a shortened position (e.g., following immobilisation after fracture or as a result of spasticity with a loss of muscle control) is more likely to develop muscle and soft tissue shortening, and is therefore at risk of contracture. If not resolved with conservative methods, it may need resolving surgically. Contracture can affect a patient's posture, activity, or hygiene, and can cause discomfort. The key to management is in preventative measures including effective positioning, seating, orthoses, and spasticity management.

## Fractures

Orthopaedic injuries can cause limitations in muscle range and power, meaning that patients may not be able to move and position themselves effectively. They may also have internal or external fixators which present a risk of infection or migration. Patients with fractures (especially spinal fractures) may also need to wear braces for certain movements which may increase the risk of pressure areas and discomfort (which can cause issues with compliance). Orthopaedic protocols will be set by surgical teams for individual patients; these may include restrictions to movement and weight bearing which may affect a patient's ability to participate and progress with rehabilitation.

## Amputation

Patients admitted to a specialist rehabilitation unit may be admitted with surgical or traumatic amputation of one or more limbs. Close work with tissue viability teams, vascular specialists, orthopaedics, and prosthetics services is vital to ensure the correct management of these patients. Correct stump management and use of pressure garments at the right time are imperative if the patient is likely to use a prosthesis in the future.

   Careful management and monitoring of patients with pre-existing prostheses is important, as muscle wasting and weight changes, linked to severe injury, may alter the fit of artificial limbs. Patients with lower limb amputations may require specific wheelchair alterations; for example, above knee amputees require wheels to be set back and may require a stump board.

## Altered blood pressure

Orthostatic hypotension, postural hypotension, or a 'postural drop' is defined as a drop of greater than 20/10 (systolic/diastolic) mm Hg within 3 minutes of changing position from lying to sitting or sitting to standing.

Risk factors include:

1. Hypovolemia (as a result of dehydration, blood loss, and anaemia)
2. Medication (beta-blockers, antidepressants, vasodilators, and Parkinson's medications)
3. Hot weather
4. Immobility (when legs become dependent and blood pools in the lower extremities)
5. Cardiovascular conditions (arrhythmia, valve disease, and vessel wall disease)
6. Neurodegenerative diseases, for example, Parkinson's disease
7. Diabetes
8. Pregnancy
9. Age 65 or over (the body's ability to react to postural changes can slow as person ages)

Orthostatic hypotension can cause dizziness and fainting and, if severe, could result in stroke due to a decrease in blood flow to the brain. Management may include: adequate hydration, review of medication, TED stockings, or abdominal binders (acting as a muscle pump), positioning patient head up/chair position in bed (acclimatises body to being in a legs-dependent position), or using a tilt table to gradually increase the patient's tolerance of more vertical postures and increased time in sitting on edge of bed before standing.

## Vestibular dysfunction

The vestibular system includes the parts of the inner ear and brain that process the sensory information involved with controlling balance and eye movements. The inner ear has three loop-shaped structures (semicircular canals) that contain fluid and have fine hair-like sensors that monitor head rotation. It also has other structures (otolith organs) that monitor linear movements. These otolith organs contain crystals that enable sensitivity to changes in movement and gravity.

If the vestibular system is damaged following a head injury, problems with balance or dizziness may be seen.

Three types of vestibular impairments commonly seen in rehabilitation settings are:

1. Benign paroxysmal positional vertigo. This is one of the most common causes of vertigo. With trauma, the crystals in the inner ear can be moved out of place, resulting in sensitivity to changes in gravity. Benign paroxysmal positional vertigo is characterised by brief episodes of mild to intense vertigo. Symptoms are triggered by specific changes in head position, such as tipping the head up or down, and by lying down, turning over or sitting up in bed.
2. Labyrinthine concussion or nerve injuries within the vestibular system are also causes of vertigo and imbalance after brain injury.
3. Traumatic endolymphatic hydrops occur when there is a disruption of the fluid balance within the inner ear.

Treatments focus on eye and head exercises, plus balance exercises, to help relieve dizziness and improve the ability to walk without losing balance. Medication and/or ear, nose, and throat specialist review may be required for persistent cases.

## Respiratory compromise

Patients with respiratory difficulties need careful positioning and mobilisation to optimise their lung function. The aim is to achieve an ideal balance between ventilation (the air getting in) and perfusion (the blood getting to the lungs), also known as V/Q match. Ideally, all patients (with or without respiratory problems) should be sat up in chair position in the bed, or sat out in a chair several times each day. Sitting up allows the abdominal contents to move down and away from the diaphragm, so that patients are able to take deep breaths more easily. The patient's physiotherapist will advise on the best position for individual respiratory issues as they may benefit from postural drainage or lying on certain sides to achieve V/Q match.

Patients who are weaning from ventilation, oxygen, or a tracheostomy should be discussed by the IDT daily to decide which goal takes priority for the day. For example, on some days weaning may be a priority and therefore therapists should not overly challenge the patient, physically or cognitively, as fatigue could be detrimental to the weaning process.

Oxygen saturations should be monitored for all patients while mobilising or exercising, where respiratory compromise is a concern, and relevant bronchodilators/medications should be given for patients at risk of bronchospasm on exercise.

## The role of the interdisciplinary team in 24-hour physical management

On admission, patients will be assessed by relevant members of the IDT to identify any physical issues, and to plan their physical management programme.

All members of the IDT can provide valuable input into the 24-hour physical management of each patient.

A patient's day will be divided into periods of activity and rest. New activities and specialist interventions are likely to be provided by the therapists; however, physical management does not stop at the end of a therapy session. Patients may carry out an independent exercise programme, or practice new personal care/domestic skills with nursing staff/carers. Once assessed as safe to do so, they will progress their transfers and mobility, either independently or with nurse/carer support, practicing with new equipment or aids. A postural management programme may provide a timetable for positioning in bed and/or for sitting out, with aims to increase tolerance of an upright position, and for progression to less supportive seating as the core strengthens and sitting balance improves. An orthotics programme will direct patients/nurses/carers to the donning and doffing of orthoses throughout the day and night. Regular turns and the use of sleep systems provide postural management overnight.

Those working with a patient outside of a therapy session can provide valuable information about the patient to the treating therapists. For example, they may pick up on skin marking or discomfort with the use of orthotics, fatigue after certain activity, or a patient's reluctance to perform tasks they are not confident with. Ensuring that everyone involved provides timely feedback will help patients to achieve their goals. Where possible, patients and their families should be provided with information about the techniques being used, in order to increase their understanding and optimise engagement. Any proposed changes to the physical management of a patient should be discussed with the patient, the rest of the IDT, and family/carers. Verbal information can be supplemented with:

1. Notices on the wall in the patient's bed space/room
2. Written guidance, ideally kept in a patient-held rehabilitation folder including:
    i. Exercise sheets for patient/carer/staff
    ii. Risk assessments/how to recognise adverse effects
    iii. Positioning guidelines
    iv. Transfer guidance
3. Demonstration to staff/family/carer
4. Photographs (e.g., of splint in place, positioning in chair, facial taping, continuous passive motion machine)

IDT members should work together, within their own professional scope and competencies, and should refer to their individual discipline's code of conduct where necessary.

## Physical management modalities
### Positioning

The importance of simple and effective positioning of patients, in *all* positions over the 24-hour period, cannot be underestimated. It is the responsibility of everyone who sees a patient to ensure that they are left in a comfortable position that will not cause them any further impairment or pain. The purpose of good positioning is to limit musculoskeletal changes, prevent pressure areas, inhibit spasticity, and enhance functional independence where possible (Bromley, 2006). Limbs should be supported in a neutral position. Patients who cannot move independently should have regular turns to prevent pressure areas and improve comfort. Positioning can be as simple as elevating a swollen limb on pillows or changing bed position, or more complex, with the involvement of outside agencies for the supply of sleep systems or specialist seating.

## Seating

Seating is traditionally assessed by occupational therapists, using pressure recommendations from the nursing team. Effective seating allows a patient optimal positioning for swallowing, stimulation/socialisation, respiration, pressure care, and functional activity. It allows for a more relaxed position than standing by providing a larger support surface, and allows for relaxation of the leg muscles alongside activation of the trunk and upper limb musculature. For those with severe trunk weakness, specialist seating can include tilt in space functions or extra supports for the trunk, head, and limbs. Timetables for sitting patients out of bed can be created in conjunction with continence planning, personal care, therapy sessions, meal times, and visiting, in order to give patients the best chance of achieving the desired amount of time spent in a chair.

## Transfers

Care teams should use the safest method of transfer possible, whilst encouraging the patient to participate in function. There are many different transfer methods, including (but not limited to) physical assistance ± walking aids, stand/transfer aids, hoists, banana board, slide boards, and slide sheets.

Transfer guidance should be provided to all IDT members, ideally prominently placed in the patient's room. This should be reviewed and updated as necessary. If care teams are struggling to transfer the patient for any reason, the therapists should be informed so that they can troubleshoot this. Manual handling guidance can be sought as per local policy. The nurse's method for transferring may be different to that used by the therapists as part of the patient's treatment session, as new transfer methods will only be handed over when it is safe to do so.

## Stretching

Patients should be assessed for stretches by a therapist, which can then be handed over to other IDT members, and the family/carers where appropriate. Some patients may be at high risk of fractures from stretching due to long periods of immobility, malnutrition, heterotopic ossification (abnormal bone formation), contractures and/or low bone density. For this reason, carers should not take it upon themselves to stretch an apparently 'tight' body part without first discussing it with the treating therapists.

## Orthoses

Orthoses (also known as splints) can be either prefabricated ('off the shelf') or bespoke, and can be made of different materials. They are provided to increase or maintain range and reduce spasticity (often used in conjunction with medication or botulinum toxin injections). The presence of spasticity does not necessarily lead to contractures, but it can interfere with range of movement. Patients with spasticity, and little or no muscle power, are most at risk of developing contractures. Orthoses may include braces, splints, casts, slings, or supports (Figs. 5.1 and 5.2).

Splinting is a common part of treatment and 24-hour management in neurological practice. Splinting is also used in those with non-neurological injury who may be unable to protect limb posture or maintain range of movement themselves (e.g., those sedated in critical care settings), or to correct abnormal postures developed during the acute phase of illness.

Splints are typically provided by physiotherapists and occupational therapists in conjunction with orthotists, who offer prefabricated or bespoke appliances to provide support to joints with muscle imbalance (e.g., low or increased tone), prevent hyperextension, accommodate long-term changes, and/or assist with rehabilitation.

Splinting continues to be used in clinical practice for prevention and treatment of contractures, despite conflicting evidence and the need for further research. Splinting is advocated as a preventative measure for contractures (NICE, 2013), as the cost of contracture management has been estimated at £10,000 where inpatient treatment and surgery were required (Wade, 1992).

Splints and orthoses should be applied and removed as guided. Ideally, photographs of correct positioning should be provided, and the splint should be clearly labelled with left or right. Skin should be monitored for pressure areas/marking, comfort, and position. If a patient is having issues with pain, they may have increased tone and may be pulling out of the splint. The therapist who made the splint should be informed if any problems arise, and splints should be removed if there is risk to the skin. Clear plans for the amount of time a splint is to be worn should be handed over to the patient/nursing staff/carers (this is especially important in an outpatient/community setting where there will be less monitoring from trained staff).

## Taping, strapping, and support garments

These are usually provided by physiotherapists and occupational therapists and supported by the nursing team over the 24-hour rehabilitation process. Taping,

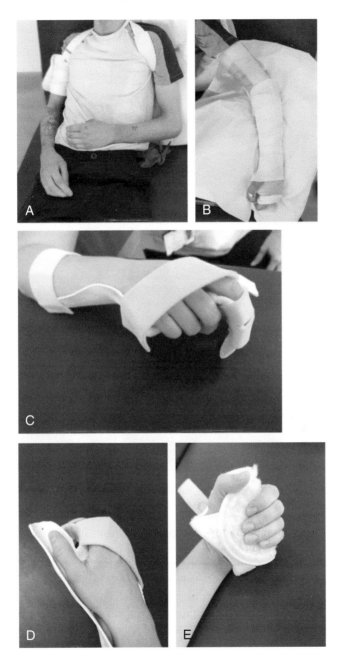

FIGURE 5.1   Upper limb orthoses and splints: (A) subluxation cuff, (B) soft and scotch splint, (C–D) thermoplastic splint, and (E) palm protector.

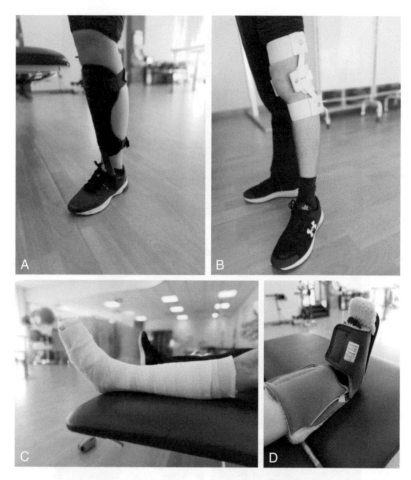

**FIGURE 5.2**   Lower limb orthoses and splints: (A) carbon fibre ankle foot orthosis, (B) Swedish knee brace, (C) soft and scotch splint, and (D) prefabricated resting splint.

position, and tensioning improve muscle engagement, support subluxed joints (Fig. 5.3), and provide proprioceptive feedback. It also allows the therapists to maintain 'hands-free' control over the position of a body part during a treatment session. Facial taping may also be advised by the speech and language therapy team to assist and give support, or to prevent, overcontraction of facial muscles, and to facilitate correct muscle posture and joint alignment. Lycra garments are used to improve proprioceptive feedback and reduce dystonic movements.

## Electrical stimulation

Electrical stimulation of muscles may be applied for reducing pain, exercise therapy, or for initiation of movement of a joint. It is only suitable for use

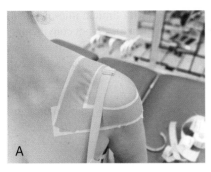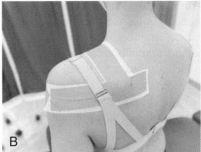

FIGURE 5.3   (A–B) Rigid taping for shoulder subluxation.

in patients with upper motor neuron injury as it stimulates muscles with an intact nerve. Contractions can be generated and coordinated to produce feedback along the neural pathways, to support neural plasticity (reorganisation of neural networks within the brain after injury), and help create functional movement. Examples of its use include facilitating grasp, walking, bladder voiding, and standing.

Functional electrical stimulation is a treatment that applies small electrical impulses to activate the peripheral nerves which lead to the muscles that have become paralysed or weakened due to damage in the brain or spinal cord. The main aim is to restore muscle function by assisting muscle recruitment while the patient practices the functional movement. Some patients rely on functional electrical stimulation for certain movements (e.g., for supporting dorsiflexion in gait), and some use it to support their recovery with a view to discontinuing use of the machine as they improve. The most common uses are with drop foot or the plegic subluxed shoulder.

Transcutaneous electrical nerve stimulation focuses on stimulating nerves with a mild electrical current, to reduce both acute and chronic pain as an adjunct or alternative to pharmaceutical analgesia.

## Constraint-induced movement therapy

The theory behind constraint-induced movement therapy (CIMT) is that when somebody has an interruption to normal nerve function in a limb, there is a learned 'nonuse' whereby people stop using the limb, yet the limb may have greater movement ability than it appears to show in everyday tasks. Following this theory, Corbetta et al. (2015) suggest that constraining the unaffected upper limb would 'force' the person to use the affected arm and movement would be improved in the affected side.

When following this programme, the constraint (usually a sling or splint) is worn for 90% of waking hours, and several hours per day should be committed to progressively more difficult exercises. A Cochrane review found that 'compared with traditional rehabilitation, CIMT is associated with limited improvements in motor impairment and motor function, but these benefits do not convincingly reduce disability' (Corbetta et al., 2015); however, CIMT is often used as an adjunct to traditional rehabilitation and is recommended within the 2013 NICE guidelines for Stroke Rehabilitation in Adults. CIMT can be difficult to put into practice as it is time consuming and requires a highly motivated and engaged patient. The use of CIMT should be guided by the patient's physiotherapist or occupational therapist and should be adhered to by all treating members of the IDT.

## Mechanical adjuncts

After lower limb trauma or surgery, some patients may benefit from the use of continuous passive motion equipment to maintain joint range. These should only be set by trained staff, but can be applied or removed by other members of staff after demonstration by the treating therapist or nurse.

## Medical management

Doctors may prescribe medication which can directly support physical management. The most commonly used are antispasticity medications and analgesics ('pain-killers'). Patients may undergo surgical intervention as part of their physical management, before or during their rehabilitation. Postoperative instructions should be clearly handed over on transfer to rehabilitation settings. More detail is provided in Chapter 2.

## Prosthetics

Prosthetics are artificial replacements of a missing body part. These are provided by prosthetists in either an inpatient or community setting and should be under regular review by all of the IDT to ensure appropriate fit and use. Prior to provision of a prosthesis, the wound must be managed as per local protocols and policies, otherwise the limb may not be able to accommodate a prosthesis and a patient's function may be decreased.

## Environmental adjustments

Simple adjustments to the environment can make a big difference to a patient's independence and therapeutic gains. Patients with spatial neglect should be encouraged to look to the affected side, and it is worth asking visitors to sit on this side for this reason. Televisions should be able to be moved freely around the patient's bedside so that their neck does not remain in a fixed position for large periods of time. To improve independence, items should be left within reach of a patient's nonaffected limb.

Patients who are particularly affected by noise and overstimulation should be in a side room where possible, to allow periods of rest. They should not be overwhelmed with personal belongings or visitors, as this will add to their fatigue, which in turn will affect their ability to participate in therapy.

## Assistive technology

Assistive technology teams usually comprise engineers and occupational therapists who assess and provide technology for patients with profound/complex physical disabilities who are unable to use standard controls (e.g., hospital call bells, TV remote, light switches, opening blinds, controlling temperature, changing bed position, and answering the door) to function independently, or are unable to communicate effectively. This service can be provided both in hospital and in the home. Assistive controls are only suitable for patients who are cognitively and physically able to use the equipment provided.

## Discharge planning

On discharge from hospital, careful planning is needed to ensure that patients are safe in their own environment, whether they are discharged home or to another care facility. In order to promote independence and/or reduce the risk of falls, this may involve the following:

1. Grab rails
2. Assistive technology
3. Equipment to support activities of daily living (e.g., perching stool, toilet seat/chair/bed raise, and kitchen trolley)
4. Ramps
5. Mobility aids
6. Stairlifts
7. Widening of doors
8. Wheelchair/specialist seating provision
9. Hospital bed/mattress
10. Visual aids
11. Hoisting equipment
12. Adaptive cutlery
13. Falls alarms

Patients/carers should know who to contact if there is a deterioration in their physical condition and should be shown how to care for their physical problems. Patients are often discharged before they are physically optimised when community therapy input can be provided to continue goal-focused work. Patients with complex injuries may require readmission to inpatient rehabilitation at a later date (e.g., following further surgery or a change in their condition).

## Summary

An interdisciplinary approach to physical and postural management is essential for those undergoing rehabilitation for physical impairment. A culture of 24-hour care should be promoted to ensure that patients reach their potential, and do so in as short a time possible. This chapter has described in detail many of the physical issues patients may encounter after complex injury or illness, and the consequences of neglecting these. It has also described some of the specific interventions that may be employed by the IDT to manage physical problems.

Box 5.1 provides a summary of the benefits patients may see if provided with an effective interdisciplinary 24-hour physical management programme.

---

**Box 5.1 Benefits of good postural and physical management**
- Prevention of soft tissue shortening and contractures
- Reduced risk of pressure sores
- Allows the patient to reach optimal level of mobility and activity
- Improved manual handling techniques (decrease risk of injury to patient, staff, or carer)
- Improved patient accessibility, reduced care needs
- Improved maintenance of hygiene (e.g., able to open hands to cut nails, clean under armpits)
- Allows the patient to be seated
- Reduced risk of chest infection
- Stimulation of digestive system
- Improved position for feeding
- Reduction of postural hypotension
- Social engagement
- Better environmental stimulation
- Improved positioning for functional tasks
- Improved healing position for fractures
- Reduced risk of osteoporosis if able to weightbear
- Improved patient awareness of affected limb
- Improved comfort
- Improved mood
- Improved sleep
- Normalisation of daily routine

**Reflective questions**

1. After reading this chapter, what do you think are the risks associated with poor physical management?
2. Which members of the IDT do you think are responsible for the physical management of a patient?
3. What might the differences be between treating a patient on the intensive care unit compared to a rehabilitation unit?
4. What difficulties might you encounter when implementing a physical management programme in a community setting?
5. How might the physical management of a patient with a progressive condition differ from that of someone with complex musculoskeletal injuries following a road traffic collision?
6. What issues might you face with a patient with severe cognitive difficulties when trying to implement a physical management programme?

# References

Ataxia UK (2014). Ataxia: what's that? Available at: https://www.ataxia.org.uk/Handlers/Download. ashx?IDMF=df6e8227-a49e-44da-910d-efc4b10ffbb7. Accessed June 1, 2017.

Boyraz, I., Uysal, H., Koc, B., Sarman, H., 2015. Clonus: definition, mechanism, treatment. Medicinski Glasnik (Zenica) 12 (1), 19–26.

Bromley, I., 2006. Tetraplegia and Paraplegia, sixth ed. Churchill Livingstone, London.

Corbetta, D., Sirtori, V., Castellini, G., Moja, L., Gatti, R., 2015. Constraint-induced movement therapy for upper extremities in people with stroke. Cochrane Database Syst. Rev. 2015 (10), CD004433. doi:10.1002/14651858.CD004433.pub3.

Hilder, J.M., Rymer, Z.W., 1999. A stimulation study of reflex instability in spasticity: origins of clonus. IEEE Trans. Rehab. Eng. 7 (3), 327–340.

Li, K., Malhotra, P.A., 2015. Spatial neglect. Pract. Neurol. 15 (5), 333–339.

NICE (2013). Stroke rehabilitation in adults clinical guideline [CG162].

Pandyan, A., Gregoric, M., Barnes, M., Wood, D.E., van Wijck, F., Burridge, J., Hermens, H., Johnson, G., 2005. Spasticity: clinical perceptions, neurological realities and meaningful measurement. Disabil. Rehab. 27, 2–6.

Parry, S., Puthucheary, Z.A., 2015. The impact of extended bed rest on the musculoskeletal system in the critical care environment. Extreme Physiol. Med. 4 (16), 1–8.

Wade, D.T., 1992. Measurement in Neurological Rehabilitation. Oxford University Press, Oxford.

Wissel, J., Manack, A., Brainin, M. (2013). Toward an epidemiology of poststroke spasticity. Neurology 80 (3 Suppl 2):S13–S19.

# Chapter 6

# Adjusting to life after illness or injury

Cara Pelser

## Chapter outline

---

## Abstract

The aim of the chapter is to explore models of adjustment following illness or injury, encourage personal reflection, and guide the reader to explore how, as professionals, we can support an individual, who has experienced a sudden change in their physical or cognitive abilities, role or relationship, adjust to a new, and potentially more challenging, way of life. This chapter will aim to explore interdisciplinary team challenges relating to adjustment, examining how important it is that the whole team takes time to understand a patient's personal narrative (or 'journey of adjustment') and facilitate positive psychological change and adaptation. The chapter also aims to consider the needs of family members, and how their worlds can change.

## Keywords

Adjustment; Acceptance; Brain injury; Illness; Anxiety; Depression; Family

---

## Aims and objectives

The aim of this chapter is not to cover everything in the literature about adjustment, nor is it an academic literature search of models, theory, or research in the field (granted, these will be alluded to throughout). Instead, this chapter aims

A Practical Approach to Interdisciplinary Complex Rehabilitation.
DOI: https://doi.org/10.1016/B978-0-7020-8276-4.00006-0

to provide a space to reflect on what adjustment means to different people and to understand how dynamic the concept can be. The chapter will also aim to guide the reader to explore how, as professionals, we can support an individual, who has experienced a sudden change in their physical or cognitive abilities, role or relationship, adjust to a new, and potentially more challenging, way of life. Throughout the chapter, examples will be provided to bring the literature to life. The first section will address models of adjustment. I ask that you bear with the theory to begin with, as the chapter builds upon this theoretical underpinning of adjustment, before moving to a more interdisciplinary team focus, and one which is likely to feel much more relatable to you as the reader. Addressing the models first will help you to understand why individuals may present with different emotional challenges, at different stages, and in different ways.

As we are all already aware, rehabilitation is unique for each individual; consequently, so too is the process of adjustment. As the title of this book and introductory chapter suggest, the interdisciplinary team (IDT) is key to successful goal setting and rehabilitation. This chapter will aim to explore IDT challenges relating to adjustment, examining how important it is that the whole team takes time to understand a patient's personal narrative (or 'journey of adjustment') and facilitate positive psychological change and adaptation.

## What do we mean by adjustment?

The experience of adjustment is subjective. It is a personal and individual experience, expressed and lived by patients and their families in many differing ways. Identifying and agreeing on a shared definition is therefore difficult to operationalise. Taking a moment to perform a quick Google search of the term suggests that adjustment is '*the process of adapting or becoming used to a new situation*'. It is simple, to the point, identifies the presence of a 'process', and suggests that one needs to become familiar and accepting of a new way of life. However, as we know, adjustment to life-changing illness or injury is not quite as straight forward as, for example, adjusting to living in a new home or changing jobs.

Within the literature, the terms 'adaptation', 'acceptance', 'adjustment', and 'coping' are often used interchangeably. This chapter will primarily use the term 'adjustment'; however, as one must adapt, cope, and accept, in order to adjust, you can quickly see how the terms begin to merge. Brennan's (2001) definition amalgamates the above terms neatly, illustrating their interchangeable nature; adjustment is '*the processes of adaptation that occur over time as the individual manages, learns from and accommodates the multitude of changes which have been precipitated by changed circumstances in their lives*'. It is not just about the ability to cope, adjustment is a psychological, social, and developmental process.

This brings us on to the next dilemma. Do we study adjustment as a set of discrete stages, which the patient navigates their way along in a linear fashion? Or do we acknowledge that adjustment is dynamic, whereby the patient is on a journey, engaging in a fluid process, with no definitive end point? Viewing adjustment as a set of 'stages' may suggest that an end point exists, where the patient is thought to be 'well-adjusted to their illness or injury'. However, through my clinical work with such patients, I have found that adjustment can be life-long and bidirectional; new challenges can present at any stage in a patient's life, and how they cope, and subsequently adjust, may be determined by many differing factors. To put it simply, adjustment as a concept is complex, yet hopefully this chapter will enable you to reflect psychologically on your practice, facilitating you to think about the emotional impact of injury or illness on a patient's rehabilitation journey and the barriers this may pose for your professional role in rehabilitation. Do not feel afraid to reflect on your personal experiences of adjustment; personal reflection can aid the learning process.

## Using models of adjustment and grief to understand emotional reactions to injury

Theoretical models of adjustment can help us to picture, literally, the complexity of the term and appreciate just how multifaceted the concept is for the patients we work with. Simplifying the concept can have both its benefits and consequences. On the one hand, sharing a simple model with a patient can help to validate and normalise emotions and feelings; but we need to hold in mind that a more complex model may be required to support a deeper professional acknowledgement of what a patient is truly experiencing.

Most people working in a health care setting have heard of the Kubler-Ross model of grief (Kubler-Ross, 1969). Inspired by her work with terminally ill patients, Kubler-Ross developed a five-stage model of grieving, encompassing the following stages: denial, anger, bargaining, depression, and acceptance. Although we are not talking about death or dying with our patients in a rehabilitation setting, we are talking about mourning the loss of an 'old self', which shares many similarities with the process of grief. Patients, and their relatives, often refer to grieving for the loss of their preinjury self or partner following life-changing illness or injury and therefore find themselves experiencing a sense of denial, anger, and depression. Despite its oversimplicity, the Kubler-Ross model has stood the test of time (most probably because it does not over-complicate an already complicated concept), and shared with patients informatively, can have huge benefits.

Fig. 6.1 is an adaptation of the Kubler-Ross model used by the Cheshire and Merseyside Rehabilitation Network. The addition of 'exploring' and 'hope', to the already established five stages, was thought to encompass more of the complexity of the journey of adjustment for patients with physical/neurological injuries. In practice, this model is shared with patients within a booklet format (Available at: https://www.cmrehabnetwork.nhs.uk/uploadedfiles/documents/Acceptance%20and%20Adjustment%20Leaflet%20final%20-%20PIP%20amended%2014%202%2017.pdf). To make the change curve more meaningful

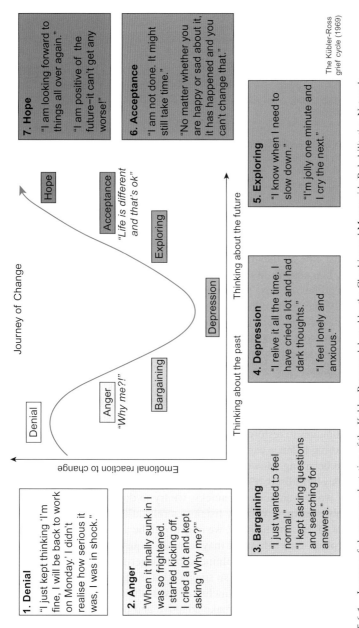

**1. Denial**

"I just kept thinking 'I'm fine, I will be back to work on Monday.' I didn't realise how serious it was, I was in shock."

**2. Anger**

"When it finally sunk in I was so frightened. I started kicking off, I cried a lot and kept asking 'Why me?'"

**3. Bargaining**

"I just wanted to feel normal."

"I kept asking questions and searching for answers."

**4. Depression**

"I relive it all the time. I have cried a lot and had dark thoughts."

"I feel lonely and anxious."

**5. Exploring**

"I know when I need to slow down."

"I'm jolly one minute and I cry the next."

**6. Acceptance**

"I am not done. It might still take time."

"No matter whether you are happy or sad about it, it has happened and you can't change that."

**7. Hope**

"I am looking forward to things all over again."

"I am positive of the future–it can't get any worse!"

Journey of Change

Emotional reaction to change

Denial

Anger
*"Why me?!"*

Bargaining

Depression

Exploring

Acceptance
*"Life is different and that's ok"*

Hope

Thinking about the past

Thinking about the future

The Kübler-Ross grief cycle (1969)

**FIGURE 6.1**  Journey of change; an adaptation of the Kubler-Ross model used by the Cheshire and Merseyside Rehabilitation Network.

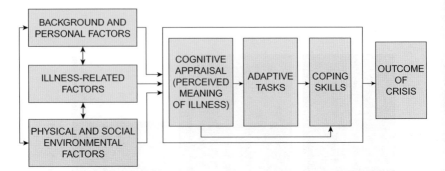

FIGURE 6.2    A conceptual model for understanding the crisis of physical illness. 'Based on Moos, R.H., Tsu,V.D., 1977. The crisis of physical illness: an overview. In: Moos, R.H. (Ed.), coping with physical illness. Plenum Press, New York'.

to the reader, patients' quotes were added to illustrate each of the stages. Patients who have read the booklet at the start of their journeys can see that change is possible, whilst those who have read/re-read the booklet towards the end can reflect on just how far they have come.

In 1977, in a chapter in the book 'Coping with Physical Illness', Moos and Tsu (1977) addressed how people who experience extreme pain and suffering miraculously manage to cope and get on with life. They set out to explore why people don't just 'give up' under the stress of physical illness and injury. The psychological, social, and developmental questions they address within their model are not particularly dissimilar to the most recent papers being published in the field today.

Moos and Tsu (1977) address the idea that as humans we strive for balance or 'equilibrium'. We want to feel psychologically and emotionally stable, therefore if something upsets this stability, we employ coping strategies and problem-solving techniques to restore balance (as we cannot remain unbalanced for very long). Restoring balance can result in a new, healthy, adaptive way of thinking, feeling, and behaving. However, if restoring balance is not possible, unhelpful strategies may be utilised, resulting in psychological decline. To provide a simple example, if we feel anxious or panicky, we try to do something to alleviate the uncomfortable feelings. We may listen to a relaxation CD and talk to someone about how we feel. Alternatively, we may avoid the anxiety, drink some alcohol, and cancel plans. One behaviour may result in 'equilibrium' being restored, the other may result in temporary calmness, but longer-term psychological distress and further decline. Moos and Tsu suggest that in this time of 'disequilibrium', or unbalance, outside influence (including us, as the professionals) could be key to supporting the individual to make adaptive and positive changes. This is an important point for us to consider in the context of rehabilitation.

Fig. 6.2 is a conceptual model of physical illness discussed by Moos and Tsu (1977). They define physical illness as a 'life crisis', to which the individual

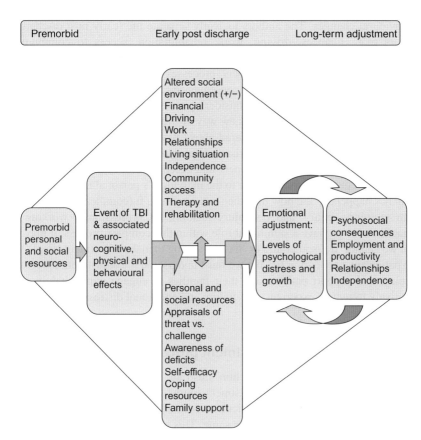

| Premorbid | Early post discharge | Long-term adjustment |

FIGURE 6.3 The experience of self in the world after ABI. 'Based on Gracey, F., Ownsworth, T., 2012. The experience of self in the world: the personal and social contexts of identity change after brain injury. In: Jetten, J., Haslam, C., Haslam, S.A. (Eds.), the social cure: identity, health and well-being. Psychology Press, London'.

applies a set of adaptive tasks and coping strategies, dependent on their own appraisal (or interpretation) of the illness. This can be impacted by the individual's background, history, previous illness, factors linked to the illness, and their physical and social environment. As you can see from studying the model, adjustment is complex and multifaceted, and many different factors can influence the 'outcome of the crisis', or how the individual adapts to life-changing illness or injury. It is unlikely that you would share this model with a patient, however, it is important to acknowledge the various dynamic factors at play.

Moving to a more recent attempt to explore the interactive factors at play in patient adjustment, Gracey and Ownsworth (2012) developed a biopsychosocial model, specifically addressing adjustment following acquired brain injury (Fig. 6.3). The model considers the impact of preinjury personal and social resources on the type of injury sustained and associated cognitive, physical, and behavioural changes. The authors logically separate the 'early post discharge' factors (e.g., finances, driving, work, rehabilitation, access to community, interpretation of the injury, and its challenges, awareness of injury, family support) from 'longer-term adjustment' processes (such as level of psychological distress/growth and psychosocial consequences; e.g., relationship breakdown and loss of independence) when considering how an individual makes sense of their new identity and adjusts to a new way of life.

It is hoped that the models offered above have not overly complicated the concept, yet instead, provided a visual display of the many processes at play when considering personal adjustment and acceptance of injury and illness. In a nutshell, adjustment comes down to the individual's personal interpretation of what has happened, and how they then make sense of it (complexly intertwined, with preinjury, injury, and postinjury factors). As professionals working in rehabilitation, we have a significant role within this complex process. It may be that we cannot 'do' something or 'fix' something to make adjustment simple for the patients we are caring for, but we must understand the adjustment processes at play, and support patients and their families to engage with rehabilitation positively to reduce experiences of failure and emotional distress.

## Factors impacting the adjustment process

As the models in the previous section illustrate, there are many factors which contribute to an individual's adjustment journey. Having worked with many patients who are experiencing difficulties with adjustment, I can say with confidence, that no two patients are the same. This gives us the extremely difficult task of understanding our patients on a personal level and adapting the way we work, listen, talk, and offer support, accordingly.

Given that, at the very least, one in four of us suffer with a mental health problem each year (McManus et al., 2009), it is very likely that patients will have a mental health history to consider. Someone struggling with depression or anxiety, just before sustaining a life-changing injury, may understandably struggle with anxiety and depression (at a heightened level) postinjury. Similarly, someone with a history of depression may quickly resort back to unhelpful coping styles and negative thinking patterns following injury or illness (Fig. 6.4).

Generally, people in modern society live fast paced, independent and highly energetic lives. Injury and illness can slow us down and create unforeseen challenges; especially for the person who is career focused, socialises, exercises in the evenings and weekends, or runs around after their children without time to 'switch off'. Adjusting to an unwanted slower pace of life may be particularly challenging for patients who are more familiar with being independent and 'on the go'. Understanding our patient's preinjury lifestyle and personal expectations is key (e.g., 'I am a dad who cooks every night', 'I work 12-hour days and I am

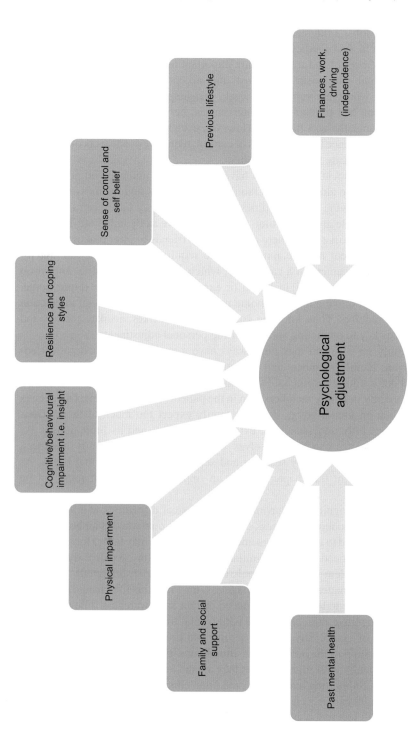

**FIGURE 6.4**  Factors affecting psychological adjustment.

good at my job', 'I run marathons for charity…'), as these expectations can play a huge role in their journey towards acceptance.

Sense of control and self-belief are important factors in determining whether an individual can positively adjust and accept life-changing injuries. An individual, who feels vulnerable, weak, and helpless, may react passively to rehabilitation and psychological intervention, believing that very little can be done to change the way they feel. However, even the most resilient patients we meet can experience feelings of loss of control, requiring positive encouragement from the health care teams around them.

Family and social support can have a significant influence on adjustment. Patients who live alone, with no family close by, may find themselves isolated and alone following injury or illness; especially if they have been in hospital for a considerable amount of time and visitors have sadly tailed off. If residual impairment is marked, and there are no family/friends to offer practical support at home, a patient may be more likely to require a transitional care bed or longer-term placement in a care home; which may have a negative impact on mental health if their original goal or expectation had been to return home. Alternatively, moving to a care home may offer the essential social interaction a patient requires. Thus, knowing your patient, their likes, dislikes, morals, and values, is key to predicting and supporting personal adjustment.

Family involvement may not always have a positive impact on patient adjustment. Family members and partners need time to adjust and accept their loved one's injuries or illness. Psychological denial and anger may be observed more overtly in family members than in the patient, which can impact a patient's rehabilitation journey (e.g., does the family expect too much of them? Does the partner fully understand the extent of the injury and its limitations?). As professionals, we can find ourselves working closely with family members, inviting them into therapy sessions and supporting their emotional needs. As discussed later in the chapter, this is an important role which must not be neglected.

A patient's cognitive, behavioural, and physical difficulties will affect their ability to adjust to injury or illness. Someone who is now wheelchair bound, who, for example, used to go to the gym and work as a joiner, may have a tough journey of adjustment ahead of them. Similarly, a patient with executive dysfunction (unable to problem solve, is impulsive and socially disinhibited), who was previously a manager of their own business, may find this life change extremely difficult to come to terms with. Reduced insight and awareness following brain injury (a cognitive difficulty linked with frontal lobe damage) can add an extra dimension of complexity to goal setting and create challenges for the team working to support the patient's transition home. The patient may not present as having difficulty with adjustment, as they are not aware of the full extent of their limitations. Supporting individuals (and often educating and supporting family) to gain insight can be a challenging task, as increasing awareness is likely to be coupled with low mood and emotional distress.

If you are a professional working with patients following life-changing illness or injury, you will know just how amazing individuals and families are when it comes to adjustment and personal resilience. People generally 'just get on with things' and make the most out of rubbish situations. However, acknowledging adjustment from the early (hospital) days is very important, as negative beliefs (such as 'I can't cope', 'I'm stupid', 'I'm not in control') can become entrenched in a person's narrative if they do not have the professional or family/social support to help them to move forward and live the best life they possibly can.

We all cope differently with life stressors. Some of us may avoid talking about the stress altogether. Others may employ a pragmatic and practical approach by trying to fix their problems or do things to overcome the stress. And some of us may be very emotional, requiring the support of others to help us to think logically at difficult times. As each of us is unique, the way we respond to stress is also unique; thus, the professional support we offer should be flexible, adaptable, and mimic the uniqueness of the patients we care for.

## The impact of psychological factors on interdisciplinary team rehabilitation

Therapeutic time (spent with physiotherapy, occupational therapy, speech and language therapy, and dietetics) is extremely precious, and therapists wish to get the most out of each session with a patient. Thus, psychological factors can sometimes be seen to 'get in the way' of successful and engaging rehabilitation. It may be good here to reflect on how you may feel in the following situation. You have recently suffered a brain injury, you are unable to walk independently, and you are emotionally overwhelmed and fatigued. You were due to go on holiday this very day with a group of friends, and you have just found out your visitor cannot make it to see you in hospital today. Your therapist is ready for you to practice walking. How do you feel?

Anxiety and low mood is reported to be more prevalent in the brain injury population, with approximately 50% of patients reporting depression during the first year after traumatic brain injury (Bombardier et al., 2010). Our patient's mood will change from day to day and hour by hour, therefore adapting session content, to meet the changing needs of the patient, may be more therapeutically significant than going ahead with a preplanned session. Spending the first 10 minutes talking to the patient, finding out how they feel that day, could result in the therapeutic rapport required to overcome future rehabilitation barriers and vitally support the patient's mental health. This may sound like common sense, but when we are pushed for time and feeling over worked, this 'common sense stuff' can be overlooked.

As you can see in Fig. 6.5, a number of psychological and neuropsychological factors can play a role in engagement with rehabilitation; not all of them warrant the intervention of a psychologist. Exploring a patient's fears, understanding their expectations, and identifying any unhelpful beliefs (such as 'I'm stupid' or

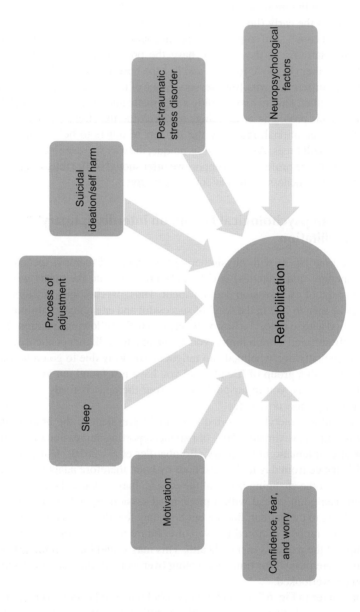

**FIGURE 6.5** Psychological factors impacting rehabilitation.

'I can't do anything right') may enhance a therapy session, and in turn therapeutic rapport. Supporting a patient to challenge a negative belief and providing positive feedback and encouragement can go a long way.

Issues with motivation can be difficult for a therapist to accept and understand for many reasons. There is a fine line between poor motivation as a result of cognitive/executive difficulties and poor motivation due to depression, fatigue, and other factors. However, whatever the origin, your role as a professional is to engage the patient the best way you can. Often family members are quick to say their loved one is being lazy, without acknowledging the role of fatigue or executive initiation problems. Therapists are key here in supporting the individual, and their family, by providing gentle encouragement and positive affirmations, or psychoeducation (if the problem appears more cognitive/brain injury related).

In an ideal NHS rehabilitation service, a team would have access to a clinical psychologist or neuropsychologist, who could support the IDT to understand the above factors and how they may impact patient engagement with rehabilitation. However, we know that a fully functioning/funded IDT can often be considered a luxury, therefore it is important that all team members take a biopsychosocial approach to rehabilitation and remain open to working dynamically across disciplines. As professionals working in rehabilitation, we all have the ability to ask how someone is feeling, and subsequently deal with a few tears; it may be that a good cathartic cry, and a listening ear, is all that is needed.

## Positive adaptation and growth

Some individuals, following life-changing injury or illness, can experience positive change (in their values, beliefs, and behaviours). Traumatic events can impact on the way an individual sees the world and the people around them, resulting in them undertaking new opportunities, improving their interpersonal relationships, increasing spirituality, and generally experiencing a greater appreciation of life (Tedeschi and Calhoun, 2004). One such example that comes to my mind is a patient who was homeless, caught up in drug and alcohol addiction, who unfortunately sustained a severe brain injury resulting in cognitive impairment. Following rehabilitation, the patient expressed that he was glad he sustained the injury as it meant that he was now alive and well. He decided to write poetry about his experiences, attended poetry events, and volunteer at the drug and alcohol rehabilitation service he used to attend as a patient.

Post-traumatic growth (PTG), as it is known in the literature, is a somewhat contentious subject. This is because there are mixed feelings about whether someone experiences *true PTG* (like I believe the patient did in the example given above) or if someone *just perceives* that they are now more compassionate and wiser. It is argued that an individual's perception of growth may be more of a coping strategy, whereby the patient is in denial about their true and honest feelings. This is something to be aware of as the two experiences (true PTG vs. the illusion of PTG) are very different psychologically (McFarland and Alvaro, 2000).

## The impact of injury or illness on the family

As we all know, injury or illness does not just affect the individual concerned. We are interpersonally connected to many other human beings who too feel the emotional impact of injury or illness. Following injury, families are at greater risk of anxiety and depression (Kreutzer et al., 1994), marital breakdown (Wood and Yurdakul, 1997), and social isolation (Brooks and McKinlay, 1983). As professionals working with families, this is something we must consider and support, if and when possible.

We must pay attention to the fact that role change occurs across the whole family network. Role strain and burden can be felt by family members (Kreutzer et al., 1992) and roles that feel forced can have a more damaging effect (Bowen et al., 2010); for example, a female partner who is now caring for her husband (helping him to wash, dress, and toilet) may feel overwhelmed and struggle to adapt to this new role which may conflict with the husband–wife relationship she is used to.

Changes in sexuality and intimacy are often observed following illness and injury for a variety of reasons; for example, role change (from partner to carer or partner to patient), cognitive impairment (poor initiation/sexual disinhibition), low mood/anxiety, brain/spinal damage, medication causing erectile dysfunction or physical impairment. Understandably, this too can cause strain on a relationship. Wives have described feeling as if they are in a child–parent relationship due to the change in roles in the household (Gosling and Oddy, 1999). Personality change can also have a burdensome effect on relationships, with male partners reporting that 'she's not the person I married' (Brunsden et al., 2015). In the same study, male partners reported 'unmet needs' and a sense of 'shared disability' with their female partner.

Lezak (1978) suggested that partners of those who have sustained an acquired brain injury find themselves living in a 'social limbo'; remaining with their partner impacts on them socially, yet abandoning the relationship leaves them open to harsh social criticism and intolerable guilt. Doka (1989) coined the term 'disenfranchised grief', a loss unacknowledged and undervalued by society. Very often family members feel a sense of grief following their loved one's injuries (especially if personality change is a consequence), yet are left 'unable' to grieve, as their loved one has not passed. Similarly, 'ambiguous loss', a type of loss experienced by many family members after a brain injury, in which the person is physically present but psychologically absent (Boss, 1999), can complicate grief and prevent closure.

We must not neglect the impact that injury or illness can have on children. They may find it difficult to understand the changes and acknowledge that a parent can no longer do what they used to do before the injury, which may, in turn, present behaviourally or emotionally at school or home. Adapting to injury or illness is a family process, and something that each family member will deal with differently, in their own way and at their own pace.

Despite the many negative consequences of injury and illness, Brunsden et al. (2015) identified positive themes within their study. Male partners reported feeling committed to their wives, never wanting to 'leave her side' and 'holding on to hope' that things will improve. Therefore, eliciting positive themes from our patients'/partners' narratives may support with motivation and gently encourage families to work together, support one another, and overcome barriers along the way.

It is so important for us, as professionals, to be aware of the positive and negative consequences of illness or injury when working with family members. They may wish to discuss and share feelings of positivity yet may need to be gently encouraged to share difficult emotions (such as grief) in times of distress. Normalising such feelings and being aware of the above literature is a key skill when working in rehabilitation settings and supporting individuals, and their families, with their acceptance journeys.

## Supporting patients and families; what can we do to help?

This concluding section may present as 'common sense' for many, however we can often neglect basic communication and listening skills when we are short on time, stressed, and feeling overworked. Listening to patients, showing compassion, and remaining nonjudgmental can support with building therapeutic rapport. Each patient's experience is entirely unique to them, and even though the patient may not present with the most limiting difficulties you have ever seen, it does not mean that they experience their challenges with any less intensity than *you* may expect them to. As we have discussed throughout the chapter, so many factors are at play when we consider adjustment to illness and injury, therefore each individual should be treated with respect, and not compared to other patients or our own preconceived ideas about how one *should* respond to a particular type of injury.

Encouraging social interaction can reduce feelings of isolation and improve patient mood. Depression can understandably interfere with participation in life activities more than the cognitive or physical sequelae of brain injury; thus, patient mental health must not be neglected and should be placed high on a team's agenda of support.

Gently encouraging and supporting patients, providing reassurance, normalising emotions (telling them it is okay to feel angry or sad), and reflecting on how far the patient has come, are key communication skills which will motivate patients, and enable them to get the best out of each therapy session. This may seem like common sense, however, it may now be a good time to reflect on your last therapy session or patient contact; what went well and what did not go to plan? Were you genuine in your praise and reassurance? Did the patient feel listened to and respected? It is entirely normal for our personalities to occasionally conflict with our patients' personalities; we do not get on with everyone we ever meet. So how do we manage such conflicting feelings? This is definitely one for supervision (or open team discussion) and should not be shied away from.

Starting a therapy session with 5 minutes of relaxation, such as deep breathing or mindfulness meditation, may support a patient to feel at ease and mentally prepared to engage with the session. This is particularly useful if the session is causing some anxiety or worry (maybe the previous session was painful, difficult, or unsuccessful). Many relaxation/mindfulness apps, videos, and music downloads are freely available and straightforward to use.

Supporting families with their adjustment narrative is extremely important for both the family and the patient. Involving family members in goal setting, inviting them into sessions, providing information and setting up family meetings will enable families to feel involved, up to date, aware of and realistic about their loved one's difficulties. It is important not to forget about the family, as they are often suffering just as much, if not more, than the individual in rehabilitation. Offering support at different stages is extremely important, as they may decline help in the early months (due to their own position in the adjustment process). Thinking about the adjustment curve (Fig. 6.1) at the start of this chapter can help with understanding when a family member may need someone to talk to.

Talking to family members about sex and intimacy may feel uncomfortable, however you will be surprised how many partners agree that acts of intimacy have declined, and that they are finding this difficult to come to terms with (especially once a patient has returned home and reality sets in). Staying on the 'taboo topics' of injury and illness, a sense of ambiguous loss/grief may feel overwhelming and difficult for family members, therefore encouraging conversation or providing a safe space to have open discussions, may need to be considered.

Finally, support groups and charities are available in the community for family members and patients to access. It is important that this information is provided in hospital, and again in community settings, to encourage those who have been through similar experiences to meet up and share stories and personal narratives of injury or illness. As professionals, it is very unlikely that we work in a service that can provide lifelong support and rehabilitation, which in some cases, would be ideal. Therefore, we must set the patient and family up with an 'emotional toolkit' from the start, which they can access when needed. A family who are made aware of the process of adjustment, the highs, the lows, and the normal feelings that can accompany life-changing illness or injury, may just be able to cope, accept, and adapt that little bit better in the future.

## Summary

This chapter has explored the topic of adjustment to illness and injury, discussing several of the models within the literature and the factors impacting emotional adjustment. Psychological factors impacting rehabilitation have been reviewed, followed by a discussion regarding how best to support individuals and their families at this difficult time. The chapter aimed to discuss the psychological literature in a way that is accessible to all those working in an IDT, or who wish to pursue a career in rehabilitation in the future. It is hoped that the reader could relate to the topics discussed, on both a personal and professional level.

### Reflective questions

Several questions to enhance learning are listed below. If you wish to create a reflective journal or logbook, this can further develop personal awareness of your practice day to day.

- What would be your personal definition of adjustment, and do you think that someone reaches an end point of 'full acceptance', or is acceptance a lifelong process or journey?
- What factors have prevented or supported you to adjust to a big change in your life?
- Thinking about a patient, is there something you could change about your practice that would support the patient in their adjustment journey? How may you implement this?
- What will you take from the chapter in terms of teamwork, and how will you support your team to think more psychologically about the patients in rehabilitation?
- What challenges have you faced when working with families? Would you do anything differently now? Have you ever worked with an individual or family with views that conflict with your own? How did you manage this?
- Now that, hopefully, you understand the terms a little better, have you come across ambiguous loss or disenfranchised grief in your personal or professional practice?

## References

Bombardier, C.H., Fann, J.R., Temkin, N.R., Esselman, P.C., Barber, J., Dikmen, S.S., 2010. Rates of major depressive disorder and clinical outcomes following traumatic brain injury. JAMA 303 (19), 1938–1945.

Boss, P., 1999. Ambiguous Loss: Learning to Live With Unresolved Grief. Harvard University, Cambridge.

Bowen, C., MacLehose, A., Beaumont, J.G., 2010. Advanced multiple sclerosis and the psychosocial impact on families. Psychol. Health 26 (1), 113–127.

Brennan, J., 2001. Adjustment to cancer – coping or personal transition? Psycho-Oncology 10, 1–18.

Brooks, D.N., McKinlay, W.W., 1983. Personality and behavioural change after severe blunt head injury: a relative's view. J. Neurol. Neurosurg. Psychiatry 46 (4), 336–344.

Brunsden, C., Kiemle, G., Mullin, S., 2015. Male partner experiences of females with an acquired brain injury: an interpretative phenomenological analysis. Neuropsychol. Rehab. 27 (6), 1–22.

Doka, K., 1989. Disenfranchised grief: Recognizing hidden sorrow. Lexington Books/D.C. Health and Com, Lexington, MA.

Gosling, J., Oddy, M., 1999. Rearranged marriages: marital relationships after head injury. Brain Injury 13 (10), 785–796.

Gracey, F., Ownsworth, T., 2012. The experience of self in the world: the personal and social contexts of identity change after brain injury. In: Jetten, J., Haslam, C., Haslam, S.A. (Eds.), The Social Cure: Identity, Health and Well-Being. Psychology Press, London.

Kreutzer, J.S., Gervasio, A.H., Camplair, P.S., 1994. Primary caregivers' psychological status and family functioning after traumatic brain injury. Brain Injury 8 (3), 197–210.

Kreutzer, J.S., Marwitz, J., Kepler, K., 1992. Traumatic brain injury: family response and outcome. Arch. Phys. Med. Rehab. 73, 771–777.

Kubler-Ross, E., 1969. On Death and Dying. Macmillan, New York.

Lezak, M.D., 1978. Living with the characterologically altered brain-injured patient. J. Clin. Psychiatry 39, 592–598.

McFarland, C., Alvaro, C., 2000. The impact of motivation on temporal comparisons: coping with traumatic events by perceiving personal growth. J. Personality Social Psychol. 79 (3), 327–343.

McManus, S., Meltzer, H., Brugha, T.S., Bebbington, P.E., Jenkins, R., 2009. Adult Psychiatric Morbidity in England, 2007: Results of a Household Survey. The NHS Information Centre for Health and Social Care. Department of Health Sciences, University of Leicester.

Moos, R.H., Tsu, V.D., 1977. The crisis of physical illness: an overview. In: Moos, R.H. (Ed.), Coping With Physical Illness. Plenum Press, New York.

Tedeschi, R., Calhoun, L., 2004. Posttraumatic growth: conceptual foundations and empirical evidence. Psychol. Inq. 9, 405–412.

Wood, R.L., Yurdakul, L.K., 1997. Change in relationship status following traumatic brain injury. Brain Injury 11 (7), 491–501.

Chapter 7

# Mental health in complex rehabilitation

Antonio Swaraj DaCosta and Jon Alan Smith

## Chapter outline

### Abstract

This chapter covers the various domains of mental health difficulties that patients admitted to complex rehabilitation may experience. It discusses the role of liaison psychiatry services within acute hospital and rehabilitation settings, legal frameworks which can be considered, and how risk towards self and others is managed.

### Keywords

Mental health; Liaison psychiatry; Neuropsychiatry; Mental Health Act; Mental Capacity Act; Psychotropic medication; Risk assessment

A Practical Approach to Interdisciplinary Complex Rehabilitation.
DOI: https://doi.org/10.1016/B978-0-7020-8276-4.00007-2

## Aims

1. To understand the roles of the different specialist mental health teams that may be involved in the management of patients with complex rehabilitation needs.
2. To understand the common types of mental illness, and the assessment and treatment options within complex rehabilitation.
3. To understand the increased complexity and risk that comes with managing patients with mental health symptoms.
4. To identify and explore best practice approaches, and how psychiatry supports the wider interdisciplinary model.

## Introduction

Patients undergoing complex rehabilitation can present with varied mental health difficulties. Some patients may have pre-existing symptoms that were undiagnosed until the new injury or illness brought them to the attention of health care professionals. Other patients may have had previous contact with mental health services; they may already have a diagnosis and require medications for their mental illness and therefore need on going follow-up. Finally, there are patients who only begin to experience mental health symptoms following illness or injury. The physical illness or injury itself may predispose an individual, without previous mental health issues, to develop mental illness, and indeed, the Holmes–Rahe life stressor scale (Holmes et al., 1967) scores 'major personal injury or illness' in the top six most stressful life events.

Over recent years, recognition of the importance for early intervention, upon identifying potential deterioration in a patient's mental health, has become a wide area of focus for health care professionals. Psychiatric diagnosis is known to impact the treatment outcome of physical rehabilitation (Silva et al., 2011). It is therefore paramount that mental health assessment is considered before, or at least alongside, the rehabilitation assessment. Ideally, complex rehabilitation services should provide the observation, monitoring, and treatment of mental and emotional wellbeing.

This chapter will explore the role of psychiatry within complex rehabilitation and provide the reader with an understanding of how its concepts influence practice within an interdisciplinary team (IDT).

## Psychiatry within a rehabilitation setting

In the United Kingdom, most mental health teams are not formally incorporated into the complex rehabilitation IDT. They would generally provide either in-reach support in the form of a liaison service, or if working with a neuroscience centre, they may be part of the neuropsychiatry unit. If the patient had previous contact with a local mental health service, efforts should aim to involve them as part of the multidisciplinary team during the rehabilitation process. Towards the end of inpatient rehabilitation, communication with the community mental health teams would be required for psychiatry follow-up. Psychiatry services should aim to work alongside the other members of the rehabilitation team to achieve outcome-orientated goals. As national policies and local services grow, complex rehabilitation will benefit from better provision of neuropsychiatry, and easy access to mental health teams.

## Liaison psychiatry

Liaison psychiatry is a specialist branch working with patients in acute hospitals presenting with psychological symptoms. They specialise in the area of medicine at the interface of physical and psychological illness. They provide specialist mental health assessment and treatment for patients in acute general hospitals. They deal with a range of problems including self-harm, adjustment to illness, and physical and psychological comorbidities. Their aim is focussed on integrated management of long-term medical conditions presenting outside formal mental health settings (Fossey and Parsonage, 2014).

The liaison team consists of a consultant psychiatrist, who, along with other doctors and advanced liaison practitioners (i.e., mental health nurses, social workers, and therapists), demonstrates an extremely flexible approach to treating the interplay between mental and physical health. Their involvement in complex rehabilitation may include general mental health assessment, crisis intervention, monitoring of the patient's mental state during inpatient rehabilitation, and working with the IDT to manage patients with risk, particularly risk to self and others.

## Neuropsychiatry

The field of neuropsychiatry is best described as an area of medicine specialising in mental health disorders which originate from injuries or illnesses affecting the nervous system. It is a growing specialty combining neurological and psychological aspects of illness. Neuropsychiatry services specialise in the diagnosis and treatment of behavioural and mental disorders caused by conditions such as epilepsy, multiple sclerosis, Parkinson's disease, functional neurological disorder, and psychiatric symptoms, where an organic cause is suspected.

Many of the specialists also have a background in working within more specialised rehabilitation units. Indeed, a complex cognitive and behavioural rehabilitation unit often has a consultant neuropsychiatrist in the IDT.

## General psychiatry

Any acute deterioration in a patient's mental state might require management in an acute inpatient psychiatric unit. In England, this may result in detention under the Mental Health Act (MHA 1983). If a patient being nursed in a rehabilitation unit is considered to lack capacity to consent to treatment due to mental illness during their admission, they may alternatively be detained under the Mental

Capacity Act (MCA). The details of these two legal frameworks are covered later in the chapter. Assessments of capacity may be supported by general psychiatry teams. Mental Health Act assessments are carried out under the expert guidance of a general psychiatry team who work across inpatient mental health units, crisis teams, and community mental health teams.

Patients with complex rehabilitation needs may also benefit from community psychiatric nurse input. A community psychiatric nurse is a specialist mental health nurse with expertise in supporting mental health recovery and monitoring outcomes, essentially providing a process of mental health rehabilitation.

With the range of mental health services available, acute and long-term management of mental illness within complex rehabilitation can be provided in various locations including acute hospitals, rehabilitation units, extended (long-term) rehabilitation units, specialised nursing/care homes, psychiatric rehabilitation units, and also within the patients' own home.

## What is 'mental health' and how do we assess it?

As health care professionals, we recognise that those patients admitted to hospital for prolonged periods of time can experience both mental and emotional distress. Commonly, patients receiving care and treatment in acute hospitals can experience symptoms of anxiety and depression, delirium, and adjustment disorders. However, of course, patients receiving care or treatment may also have pre-existing mental health diagnoses. Their presentation may also be complicated by functional disorders (symptoms with a nonorganic cause, not explained by disease) and personality disorders which may require monitoring, treatment review, or additional specialist input.

Commonly, health care professionals are encouraged to support patients to complete self-rating scales as they can be useful in screening for depression or anxiety, measuring severity, and assessing treatment outcome. These tools allow professionals to identify and monitor changes in a patient's presentation over time. There is evidence that self-rating scales, like the Hospital Anxiety and Depression Scale and the Patient Health Questionnaire-9, are valuable in identifying depression, assessing its severity, and monitoring the treatment course in primary care and in hospital settings (Hansson et al., 2009).

For those presenting with cognitive impairments, assessment tools such as the Mini Mental State Examination, Montreal Cognitive Assessment, or Addenbrookes Cognitive Examination (ACE-III or ACE-R) can be used to assess a patient's current level of cognitive functioning. These scores can provide a baseline measure of cognition following illness/injury to the brain, and be used as a reference when monitoring or reviewing a patient's progress at a later stage of rehabilitation. Families, friends, or carers can also provide health care professionals with a helpful insight into a person's cognitive function prior to the injury/illness requiring rehabilitation. For example, obtaining information about a patient's premorbid memory, orientation, recall, and language skills can allow health care professionals to understand new changes that they are otherwise unable to assess. Mental illness, both pre-existing and new, can impact cognitive state. This information can be used by health care professionals when identifying an appropriate diagnosis; however, it is important to remember that cognition can fluctuate, and additional influences can affect cognitive screening for some patients (e.g., those with visual impairment, hearing impairment, medication effects, fatigue, pain, and anxiety). Therefore it is important, at times, to interpret screening assessments with some caution.

During a mental health assessment, there are a number of areas for specific focus. This allows the mental health professional to obtain information about the patient, their characteristics, past experiences, and potential risk posed. These include their:

1. mental health symptoms and experiences
2. feelings, thoughts, and actions
3. physical health and wellbeing
4. housing and financial circumstances
5. employment and training needs
6. social and family relationships
7. culture and ethnic background
8. gender and sexuality
9. premorbid personality
10. use of drugs or alcohol
11. use of poly pharmacy
12. past experiences, especially of similar problems
13. issues relevant to them or others' safety
14. whether there's anyone who depends on them, such as a child or elderly relative
15. strengths and skills, and what helps them best
16. hopes and aspirations for the future

These specific categories capture information which is used to form a diagnosis based on the patient's presentation. A thorough assessment is needed in order to best identify treatment, support, and onwards care plans that are specific to each patient's individual needs.

## Environmental influences

Therapeutic environments are physical, social, and psychologically safe spaces that are designed to promote healing. Whilst many may find this concept 'common sense', the term therapeutic environment refers to a physical space that is set up to allow individuals to recover and/or overcome medical issues. Staff safety is also paramount in this arrangement. A simple structure that ensures staff can 'escape' when assessing a violent individual needs considering ahead of undertaking assessment. A method of ensuring the safety of lone workers, for example, carrying a telephone or alarm response system, is vital.

Therapeutic environment theory stems from the fields of *environmental psychology* (the psychosocial effects of environment), *psychoneuroimmunology* (the effects of environment on the immune system), and *neuroscience* (how the brain perceives architecture). Patients in a health care facility are often fearful and uncertain about their health, their safety, and their isolation from normal social relationships. Hospital environments can contribute to the stressful situation, and it is a recognised stress which can cause a person's immune system to be suppressed, and can dampen a person's emotional and spiritual resources, impeding recovery and healing (Smith and Watkins, 2016). The environment in which an individual receives rehabilitation can impact not only on the individual's physical health, but also on their mental health. Access to outdoor space, focussed interior design, and architecture are methods used to support a calm and relaxing place for reducing patient distress and promoting recovery. Asking families to bring in personal objects in line with infection control protocol, such as bedding, photographs, pictures, and books, can produce a more home-like atmosphere and facilitate recovery during inpatient rehabilitation.

## Psychotropic medications and their role in rehabilitation

A psychotropic (or psychiatric) medication is a licensed psychoactive drug taken to exert an effect on the chemical makeup of the brain and nervous system. They are typically made of synthetic chemical compounds. These medications can be used to treat mental illnesses. They are usually prescribed in psychiatric settings, however, can be used in primary care and acute hospital settings when prescribed by a doctor or nonmedical prescriber. These can be used once a thorough mental health assessment has been undertaken and a diagnosis formed. They can treat mood disorders, anxiety disorders, psychosis, agitation, adjustment disorders, delirium, and cognitive impairments.

Whilst there is often an identified need to prescribe medications such as antidepressants or antipsychotics, careful management of these medications is crucial within a rehabilitation setting. Medications affect people differently, and it is widely recognised that it may take some time to find the best medication for each individual. Therefore, monitoring the benefits and side effects is essential. Side effects of antipsychotic and antidepressant medications are patient-specific, however can commonly include fatigue, drowsiness or insomnia, anxiety, weight gain, dry mouth, and slurred speech. It is important to consider the consequences of these side effects on the rehabilitation process. For example, an excessively sedated patient simply will not be able to attend to the rehabilitation task at hand.

This highlights the very need for interdisciplinary working as we can use our colleagues' expert knowledge in their field to monitor effects of medication; for example, weight loss or gain may previously have gone unnoticed, however with specialist dietetic input, this would quickly be identified.

## Incidences of risk in rehabilitation

There were 6859 suicides in the United Kingdom and Republic of Ireland during 2018. In the United Kingdom, suicide rates among young people have been increasing in recent years. The suicide rate for young females is now at its highest rate on record. In the United Kingdom, men remain three times more likely to take their own lives than women, and in the Republic of Ireland four times more likely (Simms et al., 2019).

Having a psychiatric diagnosis increases the risk of suicide in a chronically disabled individual. The risk doubles in long-term hospitalised patients, in comparison to the risk present immediately after the acute neurological event (Kishi et al., 2001). A Swedish study of post stroke suicide reported that the incidence is double that of the general population (Erikson et al., 2015). There is a close association with these incidences and the rate of post stroke depression.

Risk of violence increases in the teenage years, with a peak from late teens to early 20s. Risk of violence then dramatically reduces in the late 20s, with a slow reduction until the 60s, followed by a further marked reduction. Statistics of violence within hospital settings, recorded by national nursing forums, state that there is a 10% increased risk of violence towards nursing staff during the first year of admission in the United Kingdom (RCN, 2018).

Within a rehabilitation unit, patients can be at increased risk of self-harm, depression, and violence given their prolonged period of hospitalisation and the presence of severe illness/injury. Early identification of risk factors is crucial, and it is essential to identify individuals at high risk from the outset. Risk assessment is also valuable when planning periods of home leave, because risk of suicide is known to increase once the patient leaves the hospital premises (Sakinofsky, 2014). Professionals should remain cautious and aware that risk of suicide is also known to further increase as the patient's motivation and mood improves and the patient gains insight/awareness into their disability.

## Risk assessment

Risk assessment is a key focus in psychiatry. This includes risk of self-harm or suicide, risk of aggression towards others, risk of homicide, risk from others, or other intentional or unintentional risks which may be patient-specific. It is important to not only assess current risks, but also review a patient's risk history. This allows to plan for the correct intensity and level of support being provided.

## Risk formulation

Risk formulation is based on the consideration of many factors, however is commonly categorised by current mental and emotional state, family history, previous history of harm to self, and/or others and location of injury (e.g., frontal lobes). It should be taken into account the fact that risk is dynamic, and where possible, specify factors likely to increase the risk of dangerousness, or those factors likely to mitigate violence, as well as signs that indicate increasing risk. Risk formulation brings together an understanding of personality, history, mental state, environment, potential causes and protective factors, or changes in any of these. It should aim to answer the following points.

## Risk of causing potential harm to others

The assessment and management of the risk of a person with a mental illness causing harm to another is an extremely important part of psychiatric practice. It is integral to providing safe and effective care and making decisions on transition between services. Risk cannot be eliminated, but it can be rigorously assessed and managed or mitigated, where possible. A history of violence or risk to others is vitally important, as this could help health care professionals understand the individual's premorbid behaviour which may also be impacting on the patient's current presentation. A risk assessment should also identify key factors that indicate a pattern that risk is increasing. It must also help professionals understand the behaviour, whilst trying to reduce the likelihood of the behaviour occurring, particularly as some risks are patient-specific.

## Risk of causing potential harm to self

Those who frequently self-harm are at an increased risk of suicide, whether intentionally or by misadventure, therefore it is essential to record any episodes of self-harm in a patient's history. Techniques can also help a patient in self-harm reduction; this can include using ice cubes or elastic bands as a safer alternative to cutting, scratching, biting, or burning; with this then subsequently aiming to reduce the risk of accidental suicide.

When assessing self-harm, key points to consider are:

1. Method of harming themselves intentionally such as by scratching, cutting, overdosing on medication, biting, or burning.
2. Self-harm is often liked to mental distress.
3. Everyone has their own reasons for self-harming. Some patients use self-harm as a method for coping with stressors. It is helpful to understand that self-harm is not necessarily used by patients who wish to end their life.
4. Drinking a lot of alcohol or taking drugs may increase risk of self-harm. Individuals are more at risk of death if they self-harm (accidental suicide) whilst intoxicated.
5. It is more common for young people to self-harm.

## Risk as a result of injury/illness

There are a range of additional risks that need to be considered in a complex rehabilitation patient. It is beyond the scope of this chapter to cover the details of such risk, but as part of the IDT, it is important that elements of risk are highlighted and risk management strategies implemented. These include risk of falls, risk of fire, risk from others/vulnerability, and risk of financial exploitation. More relevant to psychiatry is the risk that is triggered by personality changes following injury; for example, damage to the frontal lobe may cause patients to be disinhibited and impulsive. We cover frontal lobe injury in more details later in this chapter.

A risk management plan should promote the safety of the patient, others, or property. A clinician, having identified a risk, has a responsibility to take action with a view to ensuring that risk is reduced and managed effectively. The clinician should aim to make the patient feel safer and less distressed. Sensitive use of empathy and compassion should allow the patient to feel understood and potentially more contained.

## The Mental Capacity Act and the Mental Health Act

Within the United Kingdom, the MCA 2005 and the MHA 1983 are legal frameworks used to safeguard individuals deemed to lack capacity or require urgent care/treatment they are unable to consent to.

The MCA 2005 is designed to protect and empower people who may lack mental capacity to make their own decisions about their care and treatment. It applies to those aged 16 and over. The MCA is used when individuals suffer from cognitive impairment, brain injury, learning disability, mental illness, or lack capacity due to physical health illness such as delirium or following a stroke. It covers decisions about day-to-day things like what to wear or what to buy for the weekly shop, or serious life-changing decisions such as whether to move into a care home or have major surgery (NHS UK, 2018).

Capacity is assessed dependent on specific decisions. An example to consider here is a patient who has not consented to inpatient rehabilitation but is unable to demonstrate insight into their impairments and an understanding of the benefits of rehabilitation. This patient can be assessed under the MCA. If capacity is lacking, the patient can be detained under Deprivation of Liberty Safeguards (DoLS). This means that health care professionals can continue to provide care and treatment in the best interests of the patient. In July 2018, the government published a Mental Capacity (Amendment) Bill, which passed into law in May 2019. It replaces the DoLS with a scheme known as the Liberty Protection Safe-guards, due to come into force in April 2022. This change extends the scheme to include all settings (not just hospitals and care homes), and will include those aged 16+. It will allow NHS hospital trusts and Clinical Commissioning Groups to share the responsibility of authorising DoLS along with local authorities.

The MHA 1983, updated in 2007, informs people with mental health prob-lems what their rights are regarding assessment and treatment in hospital, treatment in the community, and pathways into hospital, which can be civil or criminal (MIND, 2018).

The MHA is, however, used at times in an acute hospital setting if a mental disorder has been identified and requires treatment. In these circumstances, a

Mental Health Act Assessment would take place which requires three professionals to complete the assessment. These three professionals are a doctor, most frequently a psychiatrist, an independent 'Section 12 approved' doctor (somebody who has received special training in mental disorders) and an Approved Mental Health Professional. Approved Mental Health Professionals are mental health professionals who have been approved by a local social services authority to carry out certain duties under the MHA.

Both acts only apply at times whereby a patient has an impairment of decision making, caused by either a mental health illness or physical health illness. They set out a legal framework for health care professionals to ensure that professionals act in the best interests of the patient when making decisions regarding treatment or care.

More commonly, in an acute hospital or rehabilitation setting, the MCA is applied, however those patients presenting primarily with mental disorder, who are considered a risk towards themselves or others, may be assessed under the MHA. The vast majority of those detained under the MHA will then be transferred for further mental health treatment to an inpatient psychiatric hospital.

## Mental health illnesses in complex rehabilitation

### Depression

Depression is the most common mental illness, with its incidence as high as one in every six individuals having experienced depression at least once in their lifetime (Kessler et al., 2005). It is characterised by the core symptoms of low mood, lack of energy, and loss of interest in pleasurable activity. Table 7.1 shows the list of symptoms seen in depression. A chronic physical health problem can both cause and exacerbate depression. Pain, functional impairment, and disability can greatly increase the risk of depression in people with physical illness, and depression can also exacerbate the pain and distress associated with physical illnesses and adversely affect outcomes, including shortening life expectancy (NICE, 2004).

Depression is approximately two to three times more common in patients with a chronic physical health problem than in people who have good physical health (NICE, 2009). The classical symptoms of depression might not be seen in all patients presenting within rehabilitation. Loss of interest and lack of concentration are more prevalent than low mood or feelings of guilt, however can also present as symptoms of cognitive decline. Variability of mood might also be evident with agitation, further complicating the picture. As patients gain insight into their condition, their risk of depression increases (Fleminger et al., 2003).

Mild to moderate depression can often be effectively treated with talking therapies, such as cognitive behavioural therapy and other psychotherapies. Antidepressants can be an effective adjunct for moderate to severe depression, but are often not the first line of treatment for cases of mild depression. Antidepressants primarily work by establishing equilibrium of neurochemicals

**TABLE 7.1 Core and other symptoms of depression.**

| Core symptoms | Somatic and cognitive symptoms |
|---|---|
| 1. Depressed mood<br>2. Loss of interest and enjoyment<br>3. Increased fatigability | 1. Reduced concentration and attention<br>2. Reduced self-esteem and self-confidence<br>3. Ideas of guilt and unworthiness<br>4. Bleak or pessimistic views of the future<br>5. Ideas or acts of self-harm or suicide<br>6. Disturbed sleep<br>7. Reduced or lost appetite |

| Mild depressive episode | Moderate episode | Severe depressive episode |
|---|---|---|
| Patients would experience two core symptoms and at least two somatic/cognitive symptoms | Patients would experience two core symptoms and at least three to four somatic/cognitive symptoms | Patients would experience three core symptoms and at least five somatic/cognitive symptoms |

Based on (WHO, 1992). ICD 10. The ICD-1–Classification of Mental and Behavioural disorders: clinical descriptions and diagnostic guidelines. Available at: https://www.who.int/classifications/icd/en/bluebook.pdf.

in the brain which are altered by the process of stress and trauma. The primary neurotransmitter implicated in depression is serotonin, and therefore the most common and widely prescribed group of antidepressants is the selective serotonin reuptake inhibitors, for example, fluoxetine, more commonly known as Prozac. Management of depression should also include the consideration of psychosocial factors; identifying stress factors (such as financial problems, difficulties at work or physical or mental abuse) and explore sources of support (such as family members and friends). The maintenance or reactivation of social networks and social activities is important.

## Anxiety

There is a close association between patients who present with depression and patients who present with anxiety. You may find that many people present with both illnesses together, with many symptoms overlapping. Due to its frequent cross occurrence the true incidence cannot be obtained, but it has been established that at least 30–40% patients after brain injury present with anxiety symptoms within the first 2 years (Osborn et al., 2016). The core anxiety symptoms include feeling scared, frightened, or nervous, sometimes without obvious cause. These feelings can then result in physical symptoms such as palpitations, sweating, breathing difficulties, stomach ache, feeling sick or nauseated, and a feeling of impending doom. These core symptoms are present in a range of diagnoses called the anxiety spectrum disorders. These include generalised anxiety disorder, panic disorder, obsessive compulsive disorder (OCD), post-traumatic stress disorder (PTSD) and adjustment disorder, which are commonly encountered in patients within rehabilitation settings.

In generalised anxiety disorder the core symptoms of anxiety are present throughout the day. This can contribute to the fatigue which a patient with a brain injury may already be struggling with. It differs from panic disorder as the latter has anxiety symptoms with episodes of panic attacks. Panic attacks are described as bursts of recurrent, sudden, intense feelings of terror without any obvious cause. Panic attacks can occur at any time and in any place without warning, thus leading to anticipation anxiety which can be present throughout the day. The person may also associate places where panic has happened previously with intense anxiety, and therefore may attempt to avoid such places.

Obsessions could be pre-existing or new features as a result of the injury. These present as anxious, obsessive ruminations which result in an urge to engage in a compulsive behaviour such as checking, cleaning, counting, and other repetitive acts. Engaging in such ritualistic behaviours relieve the underlying anxiety for the patient.

PTSD among patients with traumatic brain injury is not uncommon, despite patients not always having a clear memory of the accident. In addition to the core anxiety symptoms, they may also suffer from nightmares, flashbacks, and hyperarousal.

Adjustment disorder, as the name suggests, is a disorder that arises from maladaptive adjustment to the process of recovery. For further information relating to the process of adjustment please refer to Chapter 6 by Dr. Cara Pelser. Clinically, the disorder is diagnosed between 1 and 6 months after the trauma. Adjustment is a normal process of recovery from a stressful event, however, if during this period of adjustment the patient presents with features of depression or anxiety or both, it may be classed as a disorder and would require treatment.

Anxiety spectrum illnesses can be effectively managed with treatments similar to depression. Nonpharmacological therapies used to treat depression are also useful in the management of anxiety, namely, cognitive behavioural therapy. Most antidepressants also have antianxiety effects and therefore can be used as pharmacotherapy in the treatment of anxiety disorders. Benzodiazepines, such as diazepam, are not routinely recommended. They should only be prescribed as a short-term measure due to the risk of tolerance and dependency.

## Psychoses in rehabilitation

Most of the literature concludes that an estimate of 0.9–8.5% of people after traumatic brain injury can experience an episode of psychosis (Gurin et al., 2019). This is two to three times greater than the risk of psychosis in general population. Common psychotic experiences include hallucinations (hearing, seeing, or feeling things that are not there) and delusions (fixed false beliefs or suspicions that are firmly held even when there is evidence to the contrary). Hallucinations can be auditory or visual. When it is visual, patients describe seeing things on the ward which others cannot see, and acting on such mis-interpretation. It is essential to rule out other causes of this experience, for example, confusion due to acute infection (also called as delirium), blindness, or partial blindness caused by injury to the eye or its pathway, which can lead to visual misinterpretation. False beliefs or delusions can be of a persecutory nature, where the patient would feel threatened by people around them and might imagine others plotting a conspiracy against them. Patients with psychosis often lack insight in their illness and symptoms.

Bipolar disorder is characterised by episodes of depression and mania. Manic episodes involve elevated or irritable mood, overactivity, pressure of speech, inflated self-esteem, and a decreased need for sleep. In severe cases of depression and mania a patient might present with psychosis. It is advised that when a patient has suspected psychosis, the Mental Health Team is contacted early, as there might be a need to not only treat the patient, but also justification in using the MHA 1983.

The most effective treatment for psychosis, both with patients with brain injury and within the general population, is antipsychotic medications. These are generally dopaminergic antagonists and work by lowering the level of dopamine neurochemical in the brain which are implicated in the aetiology of psychosis.

## Frontal lobe injury

Positioned at the front of the brain, the largest of the four lobes in humans is referred to as the frontal lobe. Amongst other higher-order skills, the frontal lobes are responsible for motivation, planning, reasoning, and execution of a plan. They also play a role in personality, and injury to the frontal region of the brain can result in personality change. The frontal lobes have links with memory, in particular, working memory and attention to a task. Unfortunately, it is also the most susceptible to injury due to its location. Injury to the frontal lobes may make it difficult for the patient to initiate activity, meaning they need help in the form of prompts during rehabilitation. They may lack motivation, have difficulty planning a task and may require support executing it. The range of symptoms seen in patients with frontal lobe injury is referred to as 'dysexecutive syndrome' and more information about this can be found in Chapter 9. Often people who have known the patient before the injury would described them as 'no longer the same', having lost their old personality. They may also present as disinhibited and it might be difficult to reason with them due to the patient being overly fixated on certain demands. A neuropsychiatry team may support the wider IDT in the assessment or management of these symptoms. Often there may be a limited role for the use of medications that are aimed at specific symptoms such as agitation or impulsive behaviour. A referral to a local Brain Injury Inpatient Unit (if available) should be considered for those whose needs are predominantly in relation to dysexecutive syndrome such as behavioural or cognitive problems.

## Functional neurological disorder

Professionals working in a rehabilitation unit will commonly hear and use the terms 'functional illness' or 'functional overlay'. Despite this topic going much beyond the scope of this book, we decided that we would include a brief summary about what functional neurological disorder (FND) is, and what it means to those working in complex rehabilitation. We would recommend that the reader remains alert to this growing field, and engages in further reading on the topic, as it is something that they are likely to come across if they have not already. Local experience is that patients with FND can respond well to a rehabilitation goal-orientated approach. In the United Kingdom, there are limited complex rehabilitation units and specialist FND inpatient centres that consider rehabilitation for this group of patients. Functional illness simply means that there are no structural or systemic causes to connect a patient's presenting symptoms with a medical or organic diagnosis. The range of medical presentations FND can mimic include epilepsy, Parkinson's, and stroke. In many cases, there is a reaction to psychological processes, including past or present trauma, although it is sometimes difficult to pinpoint the actual source. The brain is thought to produce a range of symptoms and disabilities in response to psychological distress. There is increased research in this area looking at neurobiological explanations. However, a wealth of evidence supports the role of psychosocial adversities (e.g., stressful life events, interpersonal difficulties, and trauma/abuse) as significant risk factors for FND (Pick et al., 2019).

Perhaps the biggest misunderstanding around FND is that symptoms are under a patient's conscious control, and that there is always a psychological trauma (such as emotional memories following a distressing event) that has caused the symptoms. FND is often explained to patients as a psychological reaction, or as symptoms due to stress. These explanations usually fail, and result in patients feeling alienated, stigmatised, and not-believed. The main reason for the failure of such explanations is that they take a potential risk factor and turn it into the cause of the problem (Cock and Edwards, 2018).

Readers who wish to expand their knowledge of FND can access the website www.neurosymptoms.org which has a wide range of simple to understand explanations which you could utilise in your regular practice. It is vital that the psychiatry team is involved from the outset when there is a suspected diagnosis of FND, and that a team approach is implemented, involving neurology, psychiatry, and psychology, along with those providing physical therapies (physiotherapy and occupational therapy).

## Summary

This chapter has explored the role of psychiatry services within complex rehabilitation. It has provided a summary of how psychiatry services work within an interdisciplinary setting. It has explored different influencing factors, such as the mental health presentations patients may experience within rehabilitation settings, and how a holistic approach can improve the patient's journey. It is hoped the reader now has a level of understanding regarding the importance of mental and emotional wellbeing among the patients cared for in a rehabilitation unit.

### Reflective questions

Several questions to enhance learning are listed below. If you wish to create a reflective journal or logbook, this can further develop personal awareness of your practice day to day.

- Do you feel able to identify changes to a patient's mood, behaviour, or emotional wellbeing? What would be your first steps? Who would you contact?
- What factors could you change to a patient's environment to improve their health and wellbeing?
- Thinking about a patient, is there something you could change about your practice that would support the patient's mental health?
- What challenges have you faced when working with patients in your care who have emotional difficulties? Would you do anything differently now?
- Now that, hopefully, you understand the role of psychiatry a little better, how would you implement changes to your practice?

## References

Cock, H.R., Edwards, M.J., 2018. Functional neurological disorders: acute presentations and management. Clin. Med. (London). Updated 23 November 2019. Available at: https://www.fndaction.org.uk/what-is-fnd-2/. Accessed February 23, 2020.

Eriksson, M., et al. 2015. Poststroke suicide attempts and completed suicides: a socioeconomic and nationwide perspective. Neurology, 84 (17), 1732–1738.

Fleminger, S., Oliver, D.L., Williams, W.H., Evans, J., 2003. The neuropsychiatry of depression after brain injury. Neuropsychol. Rehab. 13 (1-2), 65–87.

Fossey, M., Parsonage, J., 2014. Outcomes and performance in liaison psychiatry: developing a measurement framework. Available at: https://www.centreformentalhealth.org.uk/sites/default/files/2018-09/outcomesliaisonpsych.pdf. Accessed February 18, 2020.

Gurin, L., Arciniegas, DB. Psychosis after traumatic brain injury: conceptual and clinical consideration. Psychiatric Times. Available at: https://www.psychiatrictimes.com/view/psychosis-after-traumatic-brain-injury-conceptual-and-clinical-considerations. Accessed September 24, 2021.

Hansson, M., Chotia, J., Nordstom, A., Bodlund, O., 2009. Comparison of two self-rating scales to detect depression: HADS and PHQ-9. Br. J. Gen. Pract.. Available at: https://bjgp.org/content/59/566/e283 . Accessed November 14, 2019.

Holmes, T.H., Rahe, R.H., 1967. The social readjustment rating scale. J. Psychosom. Res. Available at: https://www.psychiatrictimes.com/view/psychosis-after-traumatic-brain-injury-conceptual-and-clinical-considerations. Accessed November 2020.

Kessler, R.C., Berglund, P., Demler, O., Jin, R., Merikangas, K.R., Walters, E.E., 2005. Lifetime prevalence and age-of-onset distributions of DSM-IV disorders in the National Comorbidity Survey Replication. Arch. Gen. Psychiatry 62 (6), 593–602.

Kishi, Y., Robinson, R.G., Kosier, J.T., 2001. Suicidal ideation among patients during the rehabilitation period after life-threatening physical illness. J. Nervous Mental Dis. 189 (9), 623–628.

MIND, 2018. Mental Health Act 1983. November 2018. Available at: https://www.mind.org.uk/information-support/legal-rights/mental-health-act-1983/#.XbNc4y2ZOqA. Accessed January 30, 2020.

NHS UK, 2018, Mental Capacity Act, 10 January 2018. Available at: https://www.nhs.uk/conditions/social-care-and-support-guide/making-decisions-for-someone-else/mental-capacity-act/. Accessed November 14, 2019.

NICE. 2004. Depression in adults with a chronic physical health problem. Available at: https://www.ncbi.nlm.nih.gov/books/NBK82930/. Accessed November 2020.

NICE, 2009. Depression in adults with a chronic physical health problem: recognition and management. October 2009. Available at: https://www.nice.org.uk/guidance/cg91/chapter/Introduction. Accessed December 13, 2019.

Osborn, A.J., Mathias, J.L., Fairweather-Schmidt, A.K., 2016. Prevalence of anxiety following adult traumatic brain injury: a meta-analysis comparing measures, samples and postinjury intervals. Neuropsychology 30 (2), 247.

Pick, S., Goldstein, L.H., Perez, D.L., Nicholson, T.R., 2019. Emotional processing in functional neurological disorder: a review, biopsychosocial model and research agenda. J. Neurol. Neurosurg. Psychiatry 90 (6), 704–711.

RCN, 2018. Violence and aggression in the NHS: estimating the size and impact of the problem. Available at: https://www.rcn.org.uk/-/media/royal-college-of-nursing/documents/publications/2018/october/pdf-007301.pdf. Accessed November 2020.

Sakinofsky, I., 2014. Preventing suicide among inpatients. Can. J. Psychiatry 59 (3), 131–140.

Silva, M.A., 2011. Relationship between psychiatric diagnosis and functional outcome in physical therapy. Marquette University. ProQuest Dissertations Publishing, 2011. 3461812. Available at: https://www.proquest.com/openview/d2f6d16e9896d15c362c9b2e01f9f390/1?pq-origsite=gscholar&cbl=18750. Accessed September 24, 2021.

Simms, C., Scowcroft, E., Isaksen, M., Potter, J., Morrissey J., The Samaritans, Suicide Statistics Report, 2019. Available at: https://www.samaritans.org/about-samaritans/research-policy/suicide-facts-and-figures/. Accessed January 18, 2020.

Smith R., Watkins N., 2016. Whole Building Design Guide. Available at: https://www.wbdg.org/resources/therapeutic-environments. Accessed February 23, 2020.

WHO, 1992. ICD 10. The ICD-1 – Classification of Mental and Behavioural Disorders: clinical descriptions and diagnostic guidelines. Available at: https://www.who.int/classifications/icd/en/bluebook.pdf. Accessed November 1, 2020.

## Chapter 8

# Working with behaviour that challenges

Peter Kinsella

## Chapter Outline

**Abstract**

Behaviour that challenges can present in people who have an acquired brain injury. The term 'challenging behaviour' is subjective and lacks operational definition. There are many factors to consider from a biopsychosocial perspective as to the reasons for why it may manifest following an acquired brain injury. This chapter highlights how careful assessment of behaviour that challenges should allow for the development of a shared understanding of the behaviour to guide any subsequent intervention. Interventions should be guided by behavioural theory and principles and may also incorporate other forms of intervention. Reflections on the challenges of such work and practical pointers of support are offered in this chapter.

**Keywords**

Behaviour; Challenging; Brain injury; Psychological; Person-centred; Individual

*A Practical Approach to Interdisciplinary Complex Rehabilitation.*
**DOI: https://doi.org/10.1016/B978-0-7020-8276-4.00008-4**

## Aims and objectives

If one considers the organic, psychological, and emotional changes that can manifest as a result of brain injury/neurological trauma, the behavioural expression of any associated distress is unsurprising, but it can often present as a challenge to services. That said, the very definition of what we mean by 'challenging behaviour' is variable and often subjective. Long-standing and continued debates about 'whom' or 'what' is 'challenging' within the context of health care services has, in part, shaped legislation and guidance. Whilst much of this debate has come from learning disability services, standards, and guidance have been developed by several professional bodies (Royal College of Psychiatrists, British Psychological Society, Royal College of Speech and Language Therapists, 2007 [updated 2016];Royal College of Physicians and British Society of Rehabilitation Medicine, 2003). A move away from restrictive and reactive behavioural support frameworks has, reassuringly, been the trend in recent years (Department of Health, 2014; Positive and Proactive care— Reducing the need for Restrictive Interventions). Whilst such guidance is not specific to neurological trauma, it provides a framework for health care systems to consider person-centred, individualised assessments and interventions for behaviour that challenges (BTC). In part, this is an attempt to challenge negative, coercive system cultures. The reviews that followed the findings of institutional abuse at Winterbourne View (Department of Health, 2012), attempt to go further in highlighting the value of personalised support for challenging behaviour and how important preventative approaches are to building positive support environments (Department of Health, 2012; British Psychological Society, 2018). The term 'behaviour that challenges' shall be used for this chapter.

This is not a comprehensive or academic account of working with BTC. Rather, this chapter aims to provide an opportunity for reflection for those working with BTC and to provide an overview of the relevant topics associated with BTC. Throughout this chapter, the value of an interdisciplinary, person-centred approach to rehabilitation will be emphasised, as a guiding principle for health professionals working with BTC. It shall provide an overview of potential reasons for BTC, as well as outlining approaches to assessment and support. The emphasis of this chapter will be placed upon the behavioural effects of those with an acquired brain injury (ABI).

## What do we mean by 'behaviour that challenges'?

We have touched upon the idea that the very definition of what is perceived as a BTC is variable. It is subjective, bound by a range of factors, such as cultural norms or personal values. It can be a useful self-reflective exercise to think about the last time you experienced a situation where you were met by so-called 'challenging behaviour'. Why was it challenging? Who was being challenged? Why do you think it was challenging? Did the other person think they were being challenging? Why do you think it happened? What did you do? What did you want to change? What did *they* want to change? What was the outcome? Such reflection may help us to consider what we find challenging, and in doing so, it may open the door to developing a more holistic and formulaic approach towards BTC.

Attempts have been made to encompass these factors into a workable definition for services and service-users alike. A joint paper developed by the Royal College of Psychiatrists, British Psychological Society and Royal College of Speech and Language Therapists (Royal College of Psychiatrists, British Psychological Society, Royal College of Speech and Language Therapists, 2007) provides the following definition:

> 'Behaviour can be described as challenging when it is of such an intensity, frequency or duration as to threaten the quality of life and/or the physical safety of the individual or others and is likely to lead to responses that are restrictive, aversive or result in exclusion'.

This definition is useful in that it succinctly captures the need to consider the adverse effects that the behaviour can have on the quality of life of the individual, along with the risks it may present to others. It alludes to the idea that punitive interventions may lead to further negative experiences for the individual. Others have defined BTC as the result of a 'poor fit' between the person's needs and their environment (Emerson, 2011). These definitions provide an opportunity for us to consider BTC as a multifactorial phenomenon, as an interplay between the internal characteristics of the person and the social world in which they operate. By doing this, we widen our understanding of where the 'problem' resides, away from wholly placing responsibility on the individual, to encompass other factors also. Addressing BTC in such an individualised way is vital in reducing barriers to engagement and maintaining progress in rehabilitation (Alderman et al., 2002). Indeed, those with an ABI and significant BTC may often be excluded from the rehabilitation process and placed in inappropriate settings (Eames and Wood, 1985). There is also an overrepresentation of people with an ABI in prison settings (Pitman et al., 2015).

In the context of rehabilitation following an ABI, there are many different behaviours that can manifest which could be considered challenging (Alderman, 2007). This may include verbal or physical aggression (whether it be against other people, objects, or against themselves), disinhibited behaviour, impulsivity, dysregulated emotional control, or compulsive behaviours. Additionally, passive behaviours may be equally as challenging, such as apathy and poor motivation. Dependent on the stage of recovery, different BTC may manifest at different points in the rehabilitation journey. For example, disorientation, confusion, and agitation may result from organically driven factors during a period of post-traumatic amnesia (PTA), which will commonly improve over the days and weeks that follow from the time of injury. However, the behaviour that is exhibited during this period can be distressing for the individual, their family and the staff supporting the individual. The individual experiencing PTA may be sensitive to the effects of environmental stimulation, for example. Providing education to family members, maintaining the person's safety, and managing the level of stimulation and fatigue are likely to be key areas of intervention. Additionally, interventions may include making basic adjustments to the environment, carefully considering and managing communication styles, when interacting with the person and considering the use of some medications. When BTC manifests later in the rehabilitation journey, following emergence from any period of PTA, the behaviour is more likely to relate to residual cognitive and/or mood difficulties. This may require other approaches of support to reduce the adverse impact upon the individual and those around.

## Why does it occur?

Applied behavioural analysis theory would suggest that all human behaviour serves some purpose or function (Yody et al., 2000; Emerson, 2011). That is not to imply that the behaviour is necessarily under the intentional control of the person exhibiting the behaviour. Behaviour is goal directed and is a product of what is possible within any given situation, depending on the constraints placed upon a person's actions. Such constraints may relate to physical, communicative, cognitive, environmental, or social factors. The 'function' of a behaviour may include 'communicating' one's needs or intention, to gain attention (possibly to indicate one's needs or to seek reassurance) or to avoid/escape an aversive or unpleasant experience/stimulus. Additionally, certain behaviours may function to provide self-stimulation, possibly to alleviate boredom or to regulate emotion. It is also possible that certain behaviours exist to obtain something tangible, such as a materialistic or social reward. If we are open to the assumption that most, if not all, behaviour serves a purpose, then this opens up the opportunity to understand the potential reasons for the behaviour and to support the person with the BTC.

To expand on the idea of basic behavioural function and drive, Maslow's (1943) influential theory of human motivation may provide another way of considering the range of fundamental physiological and psychological drivers which may influence human behaviour. This theory puts forward the idea that, to be able to 'grow' (from a psychological perspective) our 'basic' needs must be attended to first, such as having access to food, water, and shelter. This, in part, provides the bedrock of security and safety upon which further development can occur. If we apply this idea to the rehabilitation process following ABI it would not be unreasonable to hypothesise that an individual's basic sense of security and safety is under threat. Potential loss of occupation, social roles, and relationships are not uncommon after such injuries; practical and existential crises can arise. Therefore, if we accept that these motivational drivers exist, then people may engage in BTC to 'recreate' a basic sense of safety and security, if their internal abilities and external social world are compromised. At a more basic level, this model also reminds us that physiological processes, such as thirst, hunger, and pain, should always be considered as potential causative or triggering factors for BTC.

In the field of ABI, there is a varying degree of reported prevalence of BTC (Alderman, 2007; Baguley et al., 2006; Sabaz et al., 2014). What is clear is that brain injury is a risk factor for BTC. The literature suggests that it is a combination of both neurocognitive components (Wood and Liossi, 2006) along with the emotional/psychological factors which combine to result in BTC following brain injury (Baguley et al., 2006).

Amongst the array of neuropsychological effects that can result from ABI, the impact of executive dysfunction appears to be particularly relevant in the context of BTC (Wood and Worthington, 2017). Impaired neuropsychological functions associated with damage to the prefrontal cortex and associated structures, along with the structures of the limbic system, appear to be particularly relevant in understanding some of the organic factors associated with BTC following ABI. Whilst integrating other regions of the brain, the frontal system primarily mediates the initiating, execution, and monitoring of goal-directed behaviour, amongst other 'higher order' skills. Impairment in this area can result in difficulties with inhibiting overlearned responses, mental flexibility, abstract thinking, and can contribute to poor decision making. Being the seat of self-monitoring, the executive system governs our ability to successfully 'update' what is working well and what might not be working so well in a given situation, allowing us to adjust our behaviour accordingly.

It is important to note that different behavioural presentations may manifest depending on the area of injury of the frontal regions of the brain. For example, an individual may present in a passive way, underpinned by apathy, and reduced behavioural 'drive', if injury occurs to the ventromedial area of the frontal brain area. In contrast, direct damage to the orbitofrontal region may result in disinhibition and impulsivity. Furthermore, where there may be significant damage to the limbic system, the medial portion of the temporal and/or connections to frontal regions, 'episodic dyscontrol' may occur (though rare), resulting in unpredictable explosive rage, which has a sudden onset and may be related to epileptiform activity (Wood and Thomas, 2013). More subtle cognitive issues may also arise from damage or disruption to the neurological systems that enable executive control of behaviour. For example, social cognition impairment may result in an individual having difficulties understanding the emotional states of others or they may fail to appropriately interpret social cues, which may act as a precipitant factor for BTC in ABI (Milders, 2019). The range of behavioural presentations potentially seen following ABI illustrates the importance of taking an individualised approach to understanding BTC, as different pathology can contribute to different behavioural presentations.

In addition to the residual cognitive deficits that may impede on behavioural regulation directly or indirectly, the psychological impact of neurological trauma should also be considered as a potential contributory factor in BTC. As explained in Chapter 6, the 'catastrophic reaction' that many people can experience following brain trauma, may result in feelings of irritability, anger, depression, and anxiety. Severe, postinjury psychiatric disturbance (which may have organic causative factors) should also be considered as part of the potential causation of behavioural disturbance postinjury (please see Chapter 7 for further information on mental health difficulties). Additional risk factors for BTC after brain injury include language difficulties (Alderman, 2007) and poor psychosocial functioning (including significant psychiatric disturbance and substance misuse) prior to the injury (Tateno et al., 2003; Sabaz et al., 2014). As discussed below, environmental factors can shape and/or maintain BTC postinjury.

In the author's experience, and consistent with literature, it is usually a combination of psychological, organic (cognitive), environmental, and premorbid factors that may combine to result in BTC. That said, we should be mindful that a behaviour (including BTC) may be serving a purpose ('function') for the individual and that ABI may change the repertoire of behaviour available to a person, as we attempt to understand and support the person presenting with the BTC.

## Assessment of behaviour from an interdisciplinary perspective

Any intervention for BTC starts with an effective individualised assessment, ideally driven from an interdisciplinary perspective. Different professional disciplines can offer unique and differing perspectives from observations of the same behaviour. As will be discussed below, a key part of a behavioural assessment is to operationalise the BTC to reduce subjectivity. Nursing staff can often be the 'eyes and ears' from an observational perspective. Whilst it sounds obvious, family/significant others and the individual themselves should also be included in this assessment process to gain their views on the BTC and information on premorbid functioning. Neuropsychological assessments can provide further understanding of an individual's cognitive strengths and areas of potential difficulty following brain injury. A thorough neuropsychological assessment would not only aid in the understanding of the more overt cognitive difficulties associated with BTC, such as executive dysfunction, but it may also identify more subtle, yet significant, cognitive changes, such as acquired problems with social cognition. Occupational therapists can also contribute to this process by assessing and understanding how cognitive impairment translates into real world function. Neuropsychiatry can provide opinion on any behavioural symptoms which may be part of a complex mental health presentation. Other medical professionals may also add to the picture. For example, exploring organic/physiological variables, such as metabolic functioning, electrolyte/hormone imbalance, infection, and/or the side effects of medication, are important factors to consider as reasons for BTC. Such factors should be investigated and potentially excluded as causes for BTC as early as possible.

As with any assessment within the rehabilitation process, behavioural assessments must be contextual. Considering the fluidity of the recovery and rehabilitation process, any changes in behaviour should alert the practitioner to consider potential reasons for this, such as infections, medication changes, or more immediate environmental/emotional stressors. Such behavioural assessments can also be vital in developing appropriate risk assessments for more harmful behaviours.

Before considering the range of methods available for assessing behaviour, there are some general points that most clinicians should consider if they are part of a team working with BTC:

1. It is always useful to make a record of the BTC, not only as part of good governance procedures, but also to aid the developing formulation.
2. When recording the behaviour, it is helpful to be as objective as possible: try to avoid emotionally laden interpretations of an event. Try not to record what you 'felt' happened but try to objectively describe the event. A useful strategy is to imagine what a camera would capture if it were recording the incident.
3. Linked to the above point is the idea that some people may avoid formally recording incidents as they worry about their role in the BTC. The important thing to remember is that we are trying to understand and support the individual presenting with the BTC, whatever those factors may be.
4. Be as specific as possible about what occurred immediately before the event and what specifically happened after the event.
5. Try not to reduce the 'person' to being defined by the BTC. Allow for separation; it is the behaviour that is challenging and therefore the behaviour we are recording.
6. Communicate between team members where appropriate. Do not ignore or keep observations to yourself if they arise. This will help to develop a shared understanding of the problem and manage potential risks.

## Methods of assessment

There are several methods of assessment. Planned and informal observation can provide naturalistic opportunities to gain an insight into the behaviour in different environments, particularly on inpatient wards. Semistructured interviews and structured questionnaires with staff members, family/carers, or the patient themselves may provide useful information about the behaviour.

Structured behavioural monitoring forms (Table 8.1) may help establish the antecedents and the consequences associated with a particular behaviour. 'ABC' charts (Cohn et al., 1994) are useful in identifying the 'antecedent' or trigger ('A') to the event, providing a description of the behaviour itself ('B'), and a record of what happened immediately after the behaviour occurred ('C', or the consequence). Neurobehavioural-specific monitoring forms have been developed. The Overt-Aggression Scale (Modified for Neurobehavioural Rehabilitation) (Alderman, Knight and Morgan, 1997) is a useful tool in defining the likely antecedents, behaviours, and consequences to behaviour more readily

**TABLE 8.1 An example 'ABC' behavioural recording chart.**

| Date/time (observer) | Situation (where did the event happen) | Antecedent (what was happening directly before the behaviour occurred?) | Behaviour (describe the behaviour that was observed) | Consequence (what happened immediately following the behaviour? |
|---|---|---|---|---|
| 2.11.20; 12:00 (PK) | Dining area. Sitting at the table | Jake had been brought from his room to the dining area. He was sitting at the table, waiting for this lunch. | Immediately after he sat down, it was observed that Jake was banging his fist against the dining table he was sat at. | Jake was asked to stop banging his fist against the table. However, this continued, and he was supported to leave the dining area and returned to his room, without any further concerns. |

seen in a neurorehabilitation environment. It provides a more objective recording of the likely presenting behaviours in neurobehavioural environments. Access to and frequent use of a range of these methods is commonplace and good practice within rehabilitation settings. Having access to a clinician (usually a psychologist) that can use this data to identify trends of the behaviour is ideal.

To explore BTC in more depth, applied functional behavioural analysis (Carr et al., 2002) may be implemented. This combines several of these assessment methods to focus on identifying the 'function' or meaning of the behaviour. Based on the idea that the behaviour is 'operating' within the environment and maintained by the consequences of the behaviour, this approach is usually best completed by a psychologist with the support of other members of the interdisciplinary team (IDT).

By combining the information collected from the assessment process with established theory, we can start to develop hypotheses about the BTC; why it may be presenting, what may be triggering it and/or maintaining it. Crucially, this 'making sense of' process may allow us to also formulate ideas about how to best intervene. This 'formulation'-driven approach should consider the unique biopsychosocial factors relevant to the person and their cultural context (Division of Clinical Psychology, 2011). Communicating this formulation with colleagues is an integral part of the process, so that there is a shared understanding of the problem.

## 'There are no triggers'

Sometimes it may be hard to identify a specific 'trigger', or indeed it may appear that the 'trigger' to the behaviour is trivial or unpredictable. Often this can be true. However, it is possible that an accumulation of several events over a short period of time can contribute to BTC. These cumulative events are referred to as 'setting events'. These events may relate to anything that increases anxiety or irritability. Consider the following hypothetical situation of a person in an inpatient rehabilitation unit who has suffered bifrontal lobe injuries following a road traffic collision. Let us imagine it is the first anniversary of the event that caused their injury. That same morning, they are informed that their therapy session has been cancelled as the physiotherapist is off sick. Later that day, they are also informed that a planned family visit has been rearranged for another date. Add to that a poor night's sleep and ongoing difficulties with psychological adjustment to their injury, the person is feeling growing resentment towards their situation. An unknowing health care assistant arrives on shift and enters the room of the patient (without knocking) to see if they would like a drink. The patient becomes instantly verbally aggressive. The health care assistant reports this behaviour as having no known 'trigger', unbeknownst to the above setting events that have accumulated to a point of resultant expressed anger. The setting events provide fertile ground for the brewing of irritability, and the fact that the staff member happened to enter the room without knocking on the door, just may have been the 'trigger' that sparked the expression of this rumbling irritability. Such an example is not untypical in the experience of the author working within inpatient neurorehabilitation environments. The most seemingly nonconfrontational (and unintentional) behaviours we produce as staff (not knocking on a patient's room door, for example) may serve to amplify feelings of worthlessness, or lack of autonomy from the patient's perspective. This highlights the importance of 'getting to know your patient'; having an awareness of what matters to them, what they value, and significant dates/anniversaries goes someway to building an individualised understanding of the people we support. It also highlights the need for effective communication between an IDT and how handovers, for example, are important forums in which we can share such information.

## Supporting the person with behaviour that challenges

Most organisations provide mandatory training on dealing with acts of aggression or de-escalation techniques and therefore, this will not be considered here. This section aims to provide an overview of some of the different approaches to managing BTC. Further to this, pharmacological approaches to the management of BTC are not covered in this chapter. There can certainly be a role for medication for these difficulties, and the reader is directed to Chapter 7 for further information.

## Behavioural approaches

Many of the approaches developed within neurorehabilitation settings are based on established behavioural principles. Any popular psychology book will inform the reader of the seminal works of behaviourists such as Skinner (1938), amongst others. Whilst the detail of such behavioural theory will not be covered here, put simply, behavioural psychology has helped us understand how behaviour can change through our experience (learning) and how behaviour can be shaped by the conditions in which that behaviour operates.

So how is this relevant to rehabilitation? It helps us consider why people may, for example, continually engage in behaviours that are seemingly challenging and 'negative', whilst also helping us consider how the behaviour is maintained. For example, a person with significant communicative and cognitive impairment may kick aggressively against their bed to elicit a response from staff. In doing so, he can 'communicate' a need for social engagement and stimulation, in an environment where proactive, attentive psychosocial care may be lacking. Although he is, unfortunately, given a verbal 'telling off' from the staff member informing him of the inappropriateness of his behaviour, as he is causing injury to himself, his desire to have some (any) form of social interaction with another person, outweighs the fact that he is potentially causing injury to himself. This is an example where there may be a suggestion that 'there is no trigger' for the BTC. The person may not be kicking out in response to any external trigger, but the behaviour is motivated by an internal drive to socially engage which does not have any obvious antecedent. Each time the staff respond, they are unwittingly reinforcing that same 'challenging' behaviour, as the 'function' of the behaviour is to gain some social attention.

Having a base knowledge of behavioural theory helps us to consider behavioural function and reflect on how the behaviours may be maintained through consequential responses. Furthermore, it is possible to 'manipulate' these factors to change or shape behaviour so that we can support the person to display an adaptive/healthy behaviour that still serves the same function as the other potentially harmful/destructive behaviour. For the example above, more proactive social interaction could be encouraged between the staff and patient, or the patient may be supported to learn to use his buzzer to initiate social interaction, which may be less destructive and harmful.

In the field of neurorehabilitation, the above-mentioned behavioural principles are often applied in line with neuropsychological theory (for example, understanding how memory and learning functions) to provide supportive behavioural interventions. Typically, two behavioural methods exist; those focussed on the *antecedents* to the behaviour and those that focus on the *consequences* to the behaviour (contingency management).

## Antecedent approaches

If we revisit the 'ABC' model of BTC (Cohn et al., 1994) as described above, we may be able to intervene at the preventative level of BTC. That is, by proactively intervening on the antecedents associated with contributing to the behaviour, we may be able to mitigate the risk of the behaviour manifesting in the first place. This could be considered the ideal method in supporting the person with

BTC within a brain injury context and this approach may be less intrusive and restrictive.

## Positive behaviour support

One example of an approach that endorses a preventative method is that of 'positive behaviour support' (Carr et al., 2002). This approach places emphasis on the antecedent factors, through functional analysis and person-centred formulation. However, it may also encompass responsive strategies to support the person's safety, incorporating principles of reinforcement. The approach is eclectic in that it draws upon strategies aimed at developing new social or communicative skills whilst also making use of social reinforcements, such as providing social attention at times when adaptive behaviours are being displayed (Ylvisaker et al., 2007). The approach attempts to look beyond the problematic behaviour itself, and towards a holistic person-centred framework, in which the individual's rights and values are central to the intervention, whilst maximising a sense of personal empowerment and choice for the individual. Collaboratively written with the individual, their family and their support team, a comprehensive and practicable document is developed to provide guidance on how to, primarily, reduce the risk of the occurrence of BTC.

## Environmental modification and managing cognitive difficulties

Making changes to the person's environment can be a useful preventative approach for some individuals. Removing stimuli which have been identified as potential triggers can be a simple yet effective preventative approach. Creating a structured, predictable environment, may help to develop a well-paced and manageable level of stimulation for those people with cognitive difficulties. A therapeutic environment in which there is an appropriate level of cognitive and social enrichment, may minimise the person becoming overwhelmed or fatigued, which can be a precipitant factor to agitation or irritability.

Basic compensatory strategies such as labelling items, providing visual cues for direction in and around the person's room, may aid those individuals with particular cognitive or sensory difficulties. Other compensatory cognitive strategies are discussed in Chapter 9 and should be considered for implementation as part of a behavioural support plan, particularly those aimed at supporting executive dysfunction. By creating this 'prosthetic environment' (Wood and Worthington, 2001), we may reduce the likelihood of the occurrence of BTC.

Whilst not specific to any situation, below lists some general ideas which can help guide preventative approaches to minimising BTC:

1. The general goal should be to improve the quality of life for the individual presenting with the behaviour along with reducing the risk to themselves or others around them.

2. This may require equipping the individual with the skills to solve their presenting problem more effectively and/or shaping their environment to better suit the needs of the person (as described above).

3. Take a whole person approach, incorporating the person's values, rights, spiritual and cultural preferences/norms, their family, and social network.

4. Taking a team approach to the BTC; being consistent with the application of the intervention is crucial. A well-developed behavioural plan may only be useful if it is consistently applied and communicated thoroughly throughout the treating team (this holds for contingency approaches also, as described below).

5. On a practical level, all team members should make it their responsibility to keep updated with any new guidelines or changes in a person's rehabilitation programme, including any guidelines on supporting behaviour difficulties. Communicate with colleagues, share, and record any observations of BTC.

6. Draw on specialist knowledge from psychology and/or psychiatry where available.

## Consequential approaches; responses to behaviour

Whilst the above preventative methods aim to work on the 'A' (antecedent) element within the 'ABC' model of behaviour, there is a long-established field of theory in the use of contingency management approaches, which focus on the responses or consequences to BTC. This is based on 'operant conditioning' principles, which is the idea that behaviour 'operates' on the environment and may be maintained/strengthened by the consequences (Skinner, 1953). 'Manipulating' these consequences/responses is therefore a key component of any contingency behavioural intervention.

Reinforcement (a response that aims to increase the frequency of a behaviour) is an example of a contingency technique. You may have heard of the term 'positive reinforcement'. This is the idea that something is 'given' when a particular behaviour occurs so that the behaviour is repeated. Giving someone a 'reward' (e.g., praise, a treat, or money) in response to desirable behaviour is an example of positive reinforcement. Some specialist neurobehavioural services use 'token economy' systems in which desirable behaviours are reinforced by tangible rewards such as tokens, which can be exchanged to purchase items. It should be noted that reinforcement does not necessarily need to be materialistic; social reinforcement (positive feedback/praise/social attention) can be equally powerful depending on the function of the behaviour. 'Negative reinforcement' is a term applied when we still want to *increase* the likelihood of a behaviour being repeated, but we do this by taking something away. For example, we are more likely to use pain-killing medication again if it is successful in 'taking away' the pain of a headache. 'Negative punishment' occurs when the goal is to *decrease* the probability of a behaviour occurring again by taking away something desirable from the person. 'Positive punishment' refers to any attempt of *decreasing* the likelihood of a behaviour being repeated by 'giving' something to the person (usually something aversive). There has been a move away from punitive punishment techniques and they are not recommended, but they are mentioned here for explanatory purposes. Careful consideration is required as to the type of technique implemented within rehabilitation services, as they pose different ethical (and potentially legal) dilemmas. The least restrictive behavioural approaches should be considered first. Indeed, consideration should always be given as to whether *any* intervention is warranted at all for any BTC as part of the decision to support the person, as determined by the ethical and risk factors associated with the BTC.

Other behavioural modification techniques exist, including 'extinction' techniques, where certain behaviours are not reinforced to reduce their effect. Withholding an expected reward or ignoring low-level (nonrisky) profanities would be examples of extinction techniques. Indeed, and as is often the case, such methods may be used concurrently. 'Differential reinforcement' techniques use both reinforcement and extinction. For example, we may want to substitute a problematic behaviour (such as swearing) with an alternative behaviour (using more appropriate language). So, we reinforce the new desirable behaviour when it is displayed (which is incompatible with the problem behaviour) but do not reinforce the behaviour that is proving challenging (such as swearing). Whilst these terms can feel a little technical, they are helpful in giving us a framework for how we can shape behaviour. It is beyond the aims of this book to go into these techniques in any detail, but the reader may want to consult with a clinical or neuropsychologist for further information/guidance.

Operant conditioning approaches may prove successful in specialised, structured neurobehavioural environments, but many have criticised the lack of generalisability within 'real world' environments. Operant conditioning approaches may not be useful for those with significant cognitive (particularly memory) impairments, as the person may not be able to learn (associate) from the consequences to their behaviour. That is why the preventative approaches may be more desirable in rehabilitation settings.

## Therapeutic relationships and communication

The importance of a person-centred approach to BTC within an IDT context cannot be overemphasised. All team members should take time to invest in the therapeutic relationship with the individual. The ever-growing demands placed on ward-based staff in health services can make it feel like a luxury to have the opportunity to simply spend time 'being' with a patient, but not every interaction has to be task orientated. Taking the time to get to know the person is of great value in building therapeutic trust and may support engagement with the rehabilitation process (Sherer et al., 2007).

Further to the above, some general points can be made with regard to developing trusting therapeutic relationships and to be mindful of how we communicate with people with cognitive difficulties, who may be in distress. Again, there is no hard rule of thumb, and we do have to be flexible in our approach to developing individualised therapeutic alliances with people. Some general ideas may include:

1. Make use of your colleagues expertise. Always liaise with speech and language therapy to gain an insight into optimising communication with those with speech or language difficulties. Speaking with a psychologist and occupational therapist may also help in thinking about how to optimally engage those with significant cognitive difficulties, such as slowed speed of thought.

2. Keep instructions simple for those with cognitive problems. Be mindful of abstract language or metaphors as they may be misinterpreted or taken literally.

3. Write things down if necessary, in words that the person will understand.

4. Provide positive feedback at every 'genuine' opportunity. Catch someone doing something well and provide feedback as soon as the behaviour was displayed.

5. If any feedback is required, it should be direct, constructive, and nonemotive. It should specify the 'behaviour' and not be critical of the person.

6. Sometimes, when providing feedback, there is a need to be firm and clear about the inappropriateness of the expressed behaviour. It can be especially important to stick to an agreed shared approach to shaping behaviour, particularly for those who may lack insight. Consistent structured feedback is coherent with building an appropriate scaffolding environment and culture (Wood and Worthington, 2001).

7. When providing feedback, try to point out something positive, but highlight what did not work and how it may be helped in the future.

8. Provide choice and options when engaging with people to maximise autonomy and independence.

9. Engage in adult-to-adult communication; avoid infantilising by using language or behaviour which may be perceived as patronising.

10. Be mindfully present during your interaction with the person. Where possible, avoid becoming too task orientated and see any interaction as an opportunity to build bridges in your therapeutic relationship.

11. Behavioural change can take time. Patience is necessary and do not become disheartened if there is not an immediate reduction (or even an increase) in BTC after an agreed plan has been implemented.

## Psychological therapy

More formal psychological therapy may be indicated where emotional adjustment difficulties exist as part of the behavioural formulation. Whilst psychological approaches to adjust to injury is covered in Chapter 6, put briefly, such interventions may provide the person with the opportunity to develop more effective coping mechanisms. Specific psychological therapy can be offered for those presenting with emotional and behavioural difficulties, such as cognitive behavioural therapy for anger management (Novaco, 1975; Medd and Tate, 2000). Such interventions can be delivered in group format or through individual sessions (Iruthayarajah et al., 2018).

It is acknowledged that psychological therapy may not be indicated for some individuals. Whilst it can be adapted, therapies such as cognitive behavioural therapy often require an ability to self-reflect and 'restructure' ones thought processes. It may be the case in the earlier stages of recovery from trauma (such as those people still in PTA, or for those with severe cognitive impairment) that other approaches are required.

It is relatively common for people to struggle with poor insight into their difficulties associated with an ABI, particularly when there are problems with executive functioning (Toglia and Kirk, 2000). This may be an additional area of intervention in the context of BTC, which can be supported by the IDT.

Finally, there are, unfortunately, some circumstances where the person's needs cannot be met in generic rehabilitation services. Whilst restrictive interventions should be avoided, high-risk behaviours may need special consideration. Admission to more specialist neurobehavioural rehabilitation services may be an appropriate course of action, which may require certain legislative procedures to be enacted. Similarly, there are situations which may put staff members at risk, and we must be mindful of knowing when it is not safe to engage or intervene.

## Reflections on learning; working with behaviour that challenges

By its very definition, working with BTC can be a stressful experience. As staff working in this field, it is important to acknowledge feelings of frustration, anger, fear, and apprehension. It is possible that our own feelings can prejudice our views of a person presenting with BTC, and potentially result in our own 'challenging behaviour'. Some may find their own personal values are incompatible with the behaviour being displayed by the individual. Others may feel incapable or unskilled in supporting certain behaviours. Furthermore, it is not uncommon for us to build negative narratives around a person with BTC, particularly if our own confidence to support the person with BTC is reduced. It is not too uncommon to hear statement such as 'oh that's just the way he is', or 'she can't change'. Whilst it is acknowledged that some people may not wish to engage with support, or they have a premorbid history that suggests unwise decision making was frequent before their injury, it is not helpful to fall into reductionist statements. This may further impede our willingness to consider the possibility for change before we have even attempted to understand and offer support.

To guard against this, a collaborative, shared team approach to BTC can be harnessed through a shared understanding between the person with BTC, and team members of the 'system' in which the behaviour manifests. There are ways in which this may be achieved; training and reflective sessions with staff could be set up, for example, possibly led by a clinical/neuropsychologist. Effective supervision of staff is imperative in supporting any difficulties in working within emotive clinical environments and should be considered a key aspect of such clinical work. 'Burn-out' and fatigue are issues which managers should be attentive to. In turn, this may help maintain ethical, compassionate, and positive approaches to supporting people who present with BTC.

## Summary

This chapter set out to increase awareness of what we mean by the term BTC, and to consider some of the reasons why people may engage in such behaviour. The assessment processes, along with a brief overview of some of the key interventions, were also considered. BTC is a complex and emotive topic. However, it is crucial that we do not lose sight of the fact that, within these complexities and challenges, there is a person; a person whose life may have unexpectedly been thrown into a sudden chaos. It is often the case that the presenting behaviour is an attempt by the person to solve a problem. By working together as an IDT, along with the person and their family/carers, we may have a greater chance of understanding and supporting the person to solve such problems. This may optimise their engagement with the rehabilitation process, thus improving their wellbeing and quality of life.

## References

Alderman, N., 2007. Prevalence, characteristics and causes of aggressive behavior observed within a neurobehavioral rehabilitation service: predictors and implications for management. Brain Injury 21 (9), 891–911.

Alderman, N., Knight, C., Morgan, C., 1997. Use of a modified version of the overt aggression scale in the measurement and assessment of aggressive behaviors following brain injury. Brain Injury 11, 503–523.

Alderman, N., Knight, C., Henman, C., 2002. Aggressive behavior observed within a neurobehavioral rehabilitation service: utility of the OAS-MNR in clinical audit and applied research. Brain Injury 16 (6), 469–489.

Baguley, I.J., Cooper, J., Felmingham, K., 2006. Aggressive behavior following traumatic brain injury. How common is common? J. Head Trauma Rehab. 21, 45–56.

British Psychological Society, Royal College of Psychiatrists, 2016. Challenging behaviour a unified approach – update. British Psychological Society, Leicester Available at: https://www.bps.org.uk/sites/bps.org.uk/files/Policy%20-%20Files/Challenging%20behavior-%20a%20unified%20approach%20%28update%29.pdf. Accessed October 6, 2021.

British Psychological Society, 2018. Positive Behavior Support. British Psychological Society, London, UK.

Carr, E.G., Dunlap, G., Horner, R.H., Koegel, R.L., Turnbull, A.P., Sailor, W., Fox, L., 2002. Positive behavior support: evolution of an applied science. J. Positive Behav. Interventions 4 (1), 4–16.

Cohn, M.D., Smyer, M.A., Horgas, A.L., 1994. The A-B-Cs of behavior change: skills for working with behavior problems in nursing homes. Venture, State College, PA.

Department of Health, 2012. Winterbourne View Hospital: Department of Health Review and Response. Department of Health, London.

Department of Health, 2014. Positive and proactive care: reducing the need for restrictive interventions. Social care, local government and care partnership directorate. Department of Health, London.

Division of Clinical Psychology, 2011. Good practice guidelines on the use of psychological formulation. British Psychological Society, Leicester, England.

Eames, P., Wood, R.L., 1985. Rehabilitation after severe brain injury: a follow-up study of a behavior modification approach. J. Neurol. Neurosurg. Psychiatry 48, 613–619.

Emerson, E., Einfeld, S., 2011. Challenging Behavior, third ed. Cambridge University Press, Cambridge.

Iruthayarajah, J., Alibrahim, F., Mehta, S., Janzen, S., McIntyre, A., Teasell, R., 2018. Cognitive behavior therapy for aggression among individuals with moderate to severe acquired brain injury: a systematic review and meta-analysis. Brain Injury 32 (12), 1443–1449.

Maslow, A.H., 1943. A theory of human motivation. Psychol. Rev. 50 (4), 370–396.

Medd, J., Tate, R., 2000. Evaluation of an anger management therapy programme following acquired brain injury: a preliminary study. Neuropsychol. Rehab. 10 (2), 185–201.

Milders, M., 2019. Relationship between social cognition and social behavior following traumatic brain injury. Brain Injury 33, 62–68.

Novaco, R.W., 1975. Anger Control: The development and evaluation of an experimental treatment. Lexington Books, Massachusetts.

Pitman, I., Haddlesey, C., Ramos, D., et al., 2015. The association between neuropsychological performance and self-reported traumatic brain injury in a sample of adult male prisoners in the UK. Neuropsychol. Rehab. 25 (5), 763–779.

Royal College of Physicians and British Society of Rehabilitation Medicine, 2003. Rehabilitation following acquired brain injury: national clinical guidelines. RCP, BSRM, London Turner-Stokes, L. (Ed.).

Royal College of Psychiatrists, British Psychological Society, Royal College of Speech and Language Therapists, 2007. Challenging behavior: a unified approach (CR144). Royal College of Psychiatrists Available at: http://www.rcpsych.ac.uk/files/pdfversion/cr144.pdf.

Sabaz, M., Simpson, G., Walker, A., et al., 2014. Prevalence, comorbidities and correlates of challenging behavior among community-dwelling adults with severe traumatic brain injury: a multicentre study. J. Head Trauma Rehab. 29 (2), 19–30.

Sherer, M., Evans, C.C., Leverenz, J., et al., 2007. Therapeutic alliance in post-acute brain injury rehabilitation: predictors of strength of alliance and impact of alliance on outcome. Brain Injury 21, 663–672.

Skinner, B.F., 1938. The Behavior of Organisms. Appleton-Century, New York.

Skinner, B.F., 1953. Science and Human Behavior. Macmillan, New York.

Tateno, A., Jorge, R.E., Robinson, R.G., 2003. Clinical correlates of aggressive behavior after traumatic brain injury. J. Neuropsychiatry Clin. Neurosci. 15, 155–160.

Toglia, J., Kirk, U., 2000. Understanding awareness deficits following brain injury. Neuro Rehabilitation 15, 57–70.

Wood, R.L., Liossi, C., 2006. Neuropsychological and neurobehavioral correlates of aggression following traumatic brain injury. J. Neuropsychiatry Clin. Neurosci. 18 (3), 333–341.

Wood, R., Thomas, R., 2013. Impulsive and episodic disorders of aggressive behavior following traumatic brain injury. Brain Injury 27 (3), 253–261.

Wood, R.L., Worthington, A., 2001. Neurobehavioral rehabilitation in practice. In: Wood, R.L., McMillan, T.M. (Eds.), Neurobehavioral disability and social handicap following traumatic brain injury. Psychology Press, Hove, pp. 133–155.

Wood, R.L., Worthington, A., 2017. Neurobehavioral abnormalities associated with executive dysfunction after traumatic brain injury. Front. Behav. Neurosci. 11, 195.

Ylvisaker, M., Turkstra, L., Coehlo, C., et al., 2007. Behavioral interventions for children and adults with behavior disorders after TBI: a systematic review of the evidence. Brain Injury 21 (8), 796–805.

Yody, B.B., Schaub, C., Conway, J., Peters, S., Strauss, D., Helsinger, S., 2000. Applied behavior management and acquired brain injury: approaches and assessment. J. Head Trauma Rehab. 15, 1041–1060.

Chapter 9

# Cognition; an assessment and rehabilitation

Nicola Branscombe, Stephen Mullin, Cara Pelser, and Wendy Owen

## Chapter outline

## Abstract

An overview of cognition is discussed and broken down into six broad areas: attention, memory, perception, apraxia, cognitive fatigue, and executive functioning. In the introduction, we will highlight the importance of a 24-hour interdisciplinary approach to managing cognitive deficits, and emphasise the importance of a person-centred approach to empower the patient and their family to self-manage any residual cognitive difficulties. The reader is signposted to other texts and resources for a more in-depth exploration of the cognitive domains highlighted within this chapter. The chapter aims to describe how a range of cognitive difficulties may impact on a person in their day-to-day life, and how cognitive difficulties can present as a challenge to the process of rehabilitation. The chapter encourages the reader to identify how they can adapt their clinical or therapeutic approach, or utilise tools, to optimise rehabilitation of patients with cognitive difficulties.

## Keywords

Cognition; Attention; Memory; Perception; Apraxia; Fatigue; Executive functioning; Brain injury

A Practical Approach to Interdisciplinary Complex Rehabilitation.
DOI: https://doi.org/10.1016/B978-0-7020-8276-4.00009-6

## Aims

1. To provide a practical introduction to cognition in the context of interdisciplinary rehabilitation.
2. To encourage a reflective, integrated approach to rehabilitation.
3. To encourage a consideration of the contribution of aspects of cognition to all areas of rehabilitation.

## Introduction

The aim of this chapter is to simplify the concept of cognition in a way that enables you, the reader, to apply theory directly to your clinical practice. We aim to do this by dividing cognition up into six broad areas: (attention, memory, perception, apraxia, cognitive fatigue, and executive functioning) to enable each area to be considered from an assessment and rehabilitation perspective. The chapter will provide examples of practice throughout, with the aim to challenge your thinking through deliberation and reflection. Throughout this chapter, and within your clinical practice, you will notice that cognitive rehabilitation cannot be addressed as a single concept (despite arranging the chapter in this reader-friendly way); therefore, please consider conceptual overlap and allow your reflective practice to move beyond single conceptual models (e.g., 'models of memory'), to considering the patient, and their cognitive difficulties, in their entirety (e.g., when discussing memory, it is inevitable that we need to consider attention and processing speed, along with many other factors). Every patient is different, every brain is unique, and therefore every injury or illness to the brain presents in its own distinctive way. Treating each patient with the same 'prescriptive' rehabilitation strategies, techniques, or tools does therefore not encompass the complexity and uniqueness of the patient sat in front of you. Interdisciplinary team (IDT) assessment should take a person-centred approach to examining cognition (exploring both pre- and post-injury factors), and collaborative goal setting should ensure that each goal is unique and tailored to the patient's needs, desires, roles, hobbies, and future aspirations.

*What is cognition?*
Cognition is highly complex. It refers to your thinking and learning skills, and your ability to perceive, understand, and explore the world around you. Cognition, as a concept, incorporates the more basic instinctual or implicit processes, as well as the complex higher-order processes that define our existence. Unfortunately, such processes are not wrapped up in cotton wool, thus cognitive skills, such as attention, memory, processing speed, and problem solving, can be affected following an injury or illness involving the brain. In rehabilitation, we are interested in whether these skills have changed. Cognitive assessments (often completed by neuropsychologists and occupational therapists) attempt to determine the preinjury (or premorbid) level of functioning (exploring education, work role, and school grades), along with the patient's cognitive strengths and

weaknesses following brain injury. When you are clear of what has 'changed' for the patient, you can help the individual to identify goals and strategies to support with these new cognitive difficulties. The image in Fig. 9.1 provides an overview of the main functions of each lobe of the brain.

Take a moment to reflect on your personal understanding of cognition before moving on. What do you look out for when talking to a patient? What questions might you ask to explore a patient's level of cognitive functioning? Would you involve family members when asking questions?

Here is a short list of some common cognitive skills which may help you to focus your initial questioning and observations when assessing a new patient following a brain injury:

1. Can the patient concentrate (sustain their attention) and divide or switch their attention?
2. Can the patient process information quickly and accurately?
3. Can the patient remember what they had for dinner the day before (long-term memory)?
4. Can the patient remember the topic of the conversation you are engaged in with them (short-term memory)?
5. Can the patient remember upcoming appointments (prospective memory)?
6. Can the patient recognise objects and understand the function of an object?
7. Can the patient name objects?
8. Does the patient know the day, date, and place (orientation), and can they recall this information when asked?
9. Can the patient plan their day, problem solve when something gets rearranged, and adapt to a new plan?

*How may a person with cognitive difficulties present?*
Take a moment to reflect on a time you have supported a patient with a brain injury. Did they present with any of the following difficulties?

1. Distracted, overwhelmed, confused.
2. Slower, in speech, thinking or movement.
3. Unable to remember what they had for lunch or who visited.
4. Difficulties with being able to sequence tasks, such as getting themselves washed and dressed, prepare a hot drink, or play a board game.
5. Unable to operate a new laptop or mobile phone.
6. Unable to use everyday objects.
7. Fatigued.
8. Angry or frustrated.
9. Unable to find their way to the café.
10. Family members reporting a change in personality, stating that their loved one is child-like or more impulsive.

For patients with cognitive difficulties, cognitive rehabilitation should be integral to their rehabilitation journey, and a team approach is required. IDTs

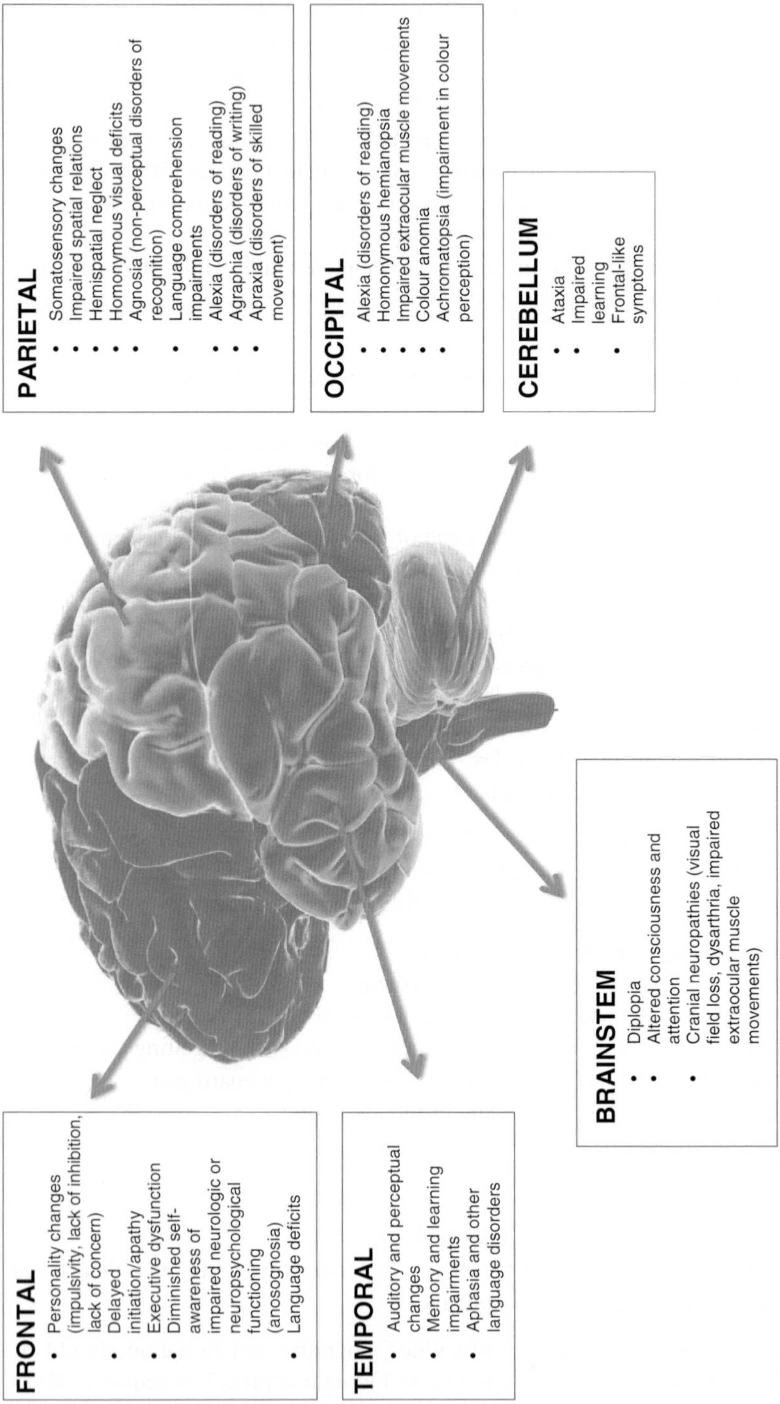

**PARIETAL**
- Somatosensory changes
- Impaired spatial relations
- Hemispatial neglect
- Homonymous visual deficits
- Agnosia (non-perceptual disorders of recognition)
- Language comprehension impairments
- Alexia (disorders of reading)
- Agraphia (disorders of writing)
- Apraxia (disorders of skilled movement)

**OCCIPITAL**
- Alexia (disorders of reading)
- Homonymous hemianopsia
- Impaired extraocular muscle movements
- Colour anomia
- Achromatopsia (impairment in colour perception)

**CEREBELLUM**
- Ataxia
- Impaired learning
- Frontal-like symptoms

**FRONTAL**
- Personality changes (impulsivity, lack of inhibition, lack of concern)
- Delayed initiation/apathy
- Executive dysfunction
- Diminished self-awareness of impaired neurologic or neuropsychological functioning (anosognosia)
- Language deficits

**TEMPORAL**
- Auditory and perceptual changes
- Memory and learning impairments
- Aphasia and other language disorders

**BRAINSTEM**
- Diplopia
- Altered consciousness and attention
- Cranial neuropathies (visual field loss, dysarthria, impaired extraocular muscle movements)

FIGURE 9.1   Image of the brain and the lobe functions.

can vary significantly across NHS Trusts and differ dependent on the setting. In an perfect, gold standard, rehabilitation setting, neuropsychology, or clinical psychology would assess and establish a patient's cognitive strengths and weaknesses based on psychometric tests and other forms of assessment (history taking/observation), including establishing a profile of their premorbid level of intellectual functioning (Casaletto and Heaton, 2017). Occupational therapists would work closely with neuropsychology to assess the impact of cognitive deficits on functional performance. They would work with patients to rehabilitate and/or compensate for these difficulties within the context of occupational goals and roles that are specific to the individual and their daily life. In addition, it is important to gain insights from the wider team about the day-to-day impact of a patient's potential cognitive difficulties. This may include discussions with nursing staff and catering staff, in addition to the patient's friends and family. It is therefore imperative that all members of the clinical team have an understanding of cognition and an awareness of how cognitive impairment can present.

*An IDT approach to cognitive rehabilitation*

An interdisciplinary model of managing cognitive rehabilitation supports a holistic 24-hour rehabilitation approach. When dealing with complex neurological presentations and medical conditions, the 'person' can sometimes get lost amongst medical diagnoses and terminology. Holistic models challenge teams to think about the patient as an individual with a unique personality; this means getting to know what is meaningful to them and what essentially 'makes them tick' (Schkade and Schultz, 1992). This approach includes considering premorbid abilities, activities, interests, and cultural background, as well as the current challenges they may be experiencing, such as pain or anxiety. All of these elements are intimately interconnected and can therefore have an impact on someone's response to rehabilitation. For example, physiotherapy can explore personal interests and hobbies to keep a patient engaged during therapy sessions, the nursing team can support phone calls to loved ones to help with feelings of loneliness and anxiety, and the catering staff can support with encouraging social communication at mealtimes.

In addition to considering the impact of the person as an individual, the environment itself can be a determining factor to the success of cognitive rehabilitation. Ben-Yishay and Diller (2008) state that if a patient's environment is organised and structured, then the cognitive demands placed on the patient are less likely to produce a 'catastrophic reaction'. Adapting the environment to promote successful outcomes will be discussed throughout the chapter and should be something which is regularly considered by the whole IDT.

Ultimately, the aim of cognitive rehabilitation is to improve functional outcomes for the patient. According to Malia (1997), cognitive rehabilitation must take a four-pronged approach; the approach needs to be structured, well-reasoned, and graded, which will help to increase patient insight, and support the patient to adjust to their new sense of self (Malia, 1997).

1. Education provided to both the patient and caregiver to help develop awareness of cognitive deficits and support with adjustment.
2. Process training ('restorative approach') to treat or retrain specific cognitive deficits. This relies on brain plasticity to aim to restore to premorbid ability. For example, a targeted task for sustained attention may include scanning through a list of letters and circling a target letter. It must be noted that there is little evidence that supports a restorative approach outside of the domain of 'attention', as improvement in one targeted task/cognitive skill has been shown to have poor generalisation to other tasks and functional outcomes.
3. Strategy training ('compensation') to teach ways to compensate for specific lost skills. Taking this approach, cognitive difficulties are compensated for by externals aids and systems, or skills that are preserved. For example, a person who has poor visual memory, but intact verbal memory, may compensate by using verbal mnemonics to encode/consolidate visual information.
4. Functional activities training using education, process, and strategy training (described above) in real life situations.

Cicerone et al. (2019) discuss the evidence base for cognitive rehabilitation in a recent systemic review, which is recommended as essential further reading. It is important to understand that cognitive rehabilitation needs to be evidence based and practice standards and guidelines need to be followed. Yet most importantly, the individual must remain at the centre of all rehabilitation goals and decisions, as the overall aim is to improve functional outcomes for the patient, to support them to return, as close as possible, to their preinjury level of functioning.

## Attention

Attention is a fundamental cognitive skill required in almost all areas of daily life, and underpinning many other cognitive functions (most importantly, memory). Deemed the 'building block of cognition' (Duncan, 2013), attention refers to how we focus on and process information in our environment. Many areas of the brain are involved in the process of 'attention', however, the frontal lobes take the majority of the workload. Poor attention, due to illness or injury to the brain, can impact the recovery/compensation of other cognitive skills, which ultimately present themselves in function (unable to attend to a conversation, follow a recipe, or focus on one task at a time).

In rehabilitation, attention is viewed as hierarchical. Imagine a pyramid were attentional processes at the top require the lower-order processes to be functioning normally. Sohlberg and Mateer (2001) clearly define each stage of the hierarchy from bottom to top as; 'focussed', 'sustained', 'selective', 'alternating/shifting', and 'divided attention/multitasking'. Therefore, according to this model, the ability to alternate attention requires intact focussed, sustained, and selective attention. This hierarchical model can allow clinicians to explore

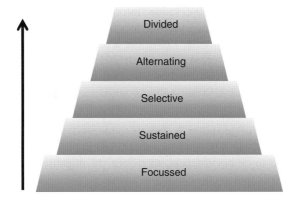

FIGURE 9.2   Cognitive hierarchy according to Sohlberg and Mateer. Based on Sohlberg, M.M., Mateer, C.A., 2001. Cognitive rehabilitation: an integrative neuropsychological approach. Guildford Press, New York.

which component of attention may be affected following brain injury using formal assessment and observation. For example, a patient who cannot sustain attention for longer than 2 minutes would find it difficult to perform a higher-order attentional skill such as dividing their attention between two tasks. Thus, rehabilitating a higher-order skill before an impaired lower-order skill would not prove useful. Fig. 9.2 demonstrates the hierarchical nature of attention according to Sohlberg and Mateer (2001).

The five levels are as follows:

1. Focussed attention is your ability to focus your attention on a specific stimuli, for example, responding to your name.
2. Sustained attention is your ability to concentrate on one activity continuously, for example, reading.
3. Selective attention is your ability to concentrate on a specific activity whilst there are other distractions in the background, for example, to attend to reading the paper whilst people are chatting in the same room, or being able to locate a person you are looking for in a busy shop.
4. Alternating/switching attention is your ability to concentrate on a task, move to a different task, and then return your concentration to the same task, for example, reading the paper, answering the phone, then returning to reading the paper.
5. Divided attention is your ability to be able to concentrate on more than one activity at the same time, simultaneously, for example, making a cup of tea whilst chatting.

Attention may appear to be a straightforward skill to address, but as with all cognitive rehabilitation, a holistic approach is required when assessing and carrying out interventions. Attention can be assessed and measured through behavioural and functional observation, information gathering, and more formally using cognitive screening tools or psychometric assessments carried out by neuropsychologists (Kinsella, 1998). For a more in-depth discussion of the complexities of attention, please refer to Fish (2017), who discusses the different models of attention and describes how attention interacts with other cognitive domains.

*Rehabilitation of attention*
The rehabilitation of attention is largely addressed through environmental changes, and the whole IDT can be aware of, and implement, such techniques. A small change to an environment, to reduce the cognitive load, can have a significant contribution to one's ability to attend.

In addition to compensatory strategies to manage attention deficits, and in line with Malia's (1997) approach, Cicerone et al. (2019) recommend direct-attention training and metacognitive strategy training to increase task performance, and generalise to function; rehabilitation techniques which are likely to be carried out by occupational therapists. It is beyond the scope of this chapter to address strategies to improve attention in their entirety, therefore further reading is suggested.

---

**Reflective questions**

Take a moment to reflect on what is happening in your environment right now? How might this environment impact on someone who has an impairment of attention?

---

Below is a list of both inpatient and community compensatory strategies that can be explored with patients with an impairment of attention.
Inpatient rehabilitation strategies:

1. Turn the radio/TV off before talking to a patient.
2. Bright lights can be over stimulating, think about the impact this may have on the patient.
3. Consider the location of a patient's bed; in a bay there are a number of distractions, both auditory and visual, compared to a side room.
4. Only one person talks at once when a patient is engaged in a task, and keep talking to a minimum until the required task is completed. This should allow the patient to engage their attention fully on what you are asking of them.
5. Minimise the amount of information that is provided at once; aim for small chunks, and then check understanding.
6. Allow a little longer for a response, the patient may be slower to process information.
7. Consider that information may need repeating.

8. Consider if the patient is being overstimulated throughout the day; they may have had the radio on, or had visitors/therapy, and therefore feel cognitively fatigued.
9. Use compensation strategies such as external cues/prompts on a piece of paper, with step-by-step instructions, to support with sequencing a task.
10. When a patient's levels of awareness is being assessed, it is important to carefully observe and record responses to different stimuli. This is discussed further is Chapter 4.

Community rehabilitation strategies (also consider adaptations of the above):

1. Educate and increase knowledge of different types of attention and how it might impact on functioning.
2. Consider if tasks can be adapted, or if compensation strategies can be used; for example, using noise cancelling earphones for certain tasks, having a prompt sheet when taking phone calls, preparing meals in advance on busy days, etc.
3. Advise the patient to complete jobs that require higher cognitive demand at times of the day the patient feels most alert.
4. Structure the day; routine and consistency is essential in rehabilitation.
5. Identify if there is anyone else who can provide support and reduce workload pressures.
6. Explore vocational rehabilitation and the impact an attentional impairment may have on returning to work, as discussed in Chapter 13.
7. Explore driving and support the patient to inform the Driver and Vehicle Licensing Agency (DVLA) about their injury and any residual cognitive impairment.

Other factors to consider when exploring and supporting attention include:

1. Pain (e.g., neuropathic or issues such as constipation)
2. Hypersensitivity
3. Fatigue
4. Types of medication
5. Psychological wellbeing

### Reflective questions

What could you change in your day-to-day practice to help support a patient's attention? Do you sometimes place too much demand (expectation) on someone who has significantly reduced attention?

**Case study: Bill**

In a hospital setting a gentleman who appears to be progressing well has just taken a cloth from his side, dipped it in some water, washed his face, then dried his face with the towel on his lap. He then picks up his comb and uses this appropriately. He is just about to look in his wash bag for his face cream, but someone pops their head into his room and says, 'Oh sorry wrong room'. Suddenly the gentleman is unsure what he was looking for in his wash bag.

1. What factors may be affecting his engagement in this task?
2. What type of attention may be impaired here?
3. What changes could be made, or rehabilitation provided?

**Case study: Anita**

A single mother at home, who has three young children, works 20 hours a week as a florist. In work she is getting distracted during a task, then when returning to the task, she notices errors have been made. She is also finding it difficult to take telephone orders. When she is home, she is finding it difficult to have conversations with the children whilst preparing the dinner.

1. What factors may be affecting her engagement in this task?
2. What type of attention may be impaired here?
3. What rehabilitation could be provided?

## Memory

Like attention, memory is an extremely complex and multifaceted cognitive process, therefore memory loss can present uniquely, dependent to some extent, on the area of the brain damaged by illness or injury. Put simply, memory is our ability to encode, store, recall, and recognise information presented both visually and verbally. It can be useful to think about memory in terms of the following three processes:

1. 'Sensory memory' is the ability to attend to relevant information, then transfer it to our short- and long-term stores (Sperling, 1960). If the information is not attended to, it is discarded.
2. 'Short-term (or working memory)' allows us to retain information temporarily, mentally manipulate this information, and then act upon this information by either retaining it or discarding it, for example, being told a phone number to dial, which will be immediately discarded if not repeated or rehearsed (Craik and Lockhart, 1972).
3. 'Long-term memory' allows us to store information for a longer period of time. If new information is to be stored as a long-term memory, it must be rehearsed or processed at a deeper level so that it can be later recalled (Squire and Zola, 1998).

Additionally, here are some of the aspects of memory that are seen and discussed within cognitive rehabilitation:

1. 'Amnesia' refers to a period for which a person has no memory. Amnesia can occur for events before or after a brain injury. Retrograde amnesia refers to the loss of memory for events immediately prior to a brain injury. Anterograde amnesia refers to the inability to form new memories for a period of time following a brain injury.
2. 'Prospective memory' allows a person to recall what they think is coming up, what to do and when to do it (Goshke and Kuhl, 1996). The ability to remember things for the future involves a certain amount of planning (and therefore executive functioning skills) in combination with memory. An example is remembering to take medications or to return phone calls.
3. 'Semantic memory' refers to knowledge and facts, whereas 'episodic memory' relates to episodes in one's life; memories of day-to-day events (Tulving, 1972). 'Autobiographical memory' can consist of semantic and episodic information and relates to personal experiences and personal knowledge.
4. 'Auditory memory' refers to memory for information which has been heard, for example, song lyrics, or the content of a conversation.
5. 'Visual memory' refers to memory for information which has been seen, for example, pictures or written words.
6. 'Recall' is the retrieval of information without a cue (free-recall), for example, when describing a picture that has previously been seen. 'Recognition' is awareness that a stimulus has been encountered before (i.e., a sense of familiarity). Recognition therefore requires a cue or prompt to work upon, for example, when indicating whether, or not, a certain picture has been seen before? (Hollingworth, 1913).
7. 'Consolidation' refers to the process by which memory for certain information, which has recently been experienced, is strengthened over a period of time following the experience. Without consolidation, information will fade from memory (Nadel and Moscovitch, 1997).

*Memory as information processing*
Memory can be conceptualised as the movement of information into the cognitive system, its storage within the system, and its subsequent retrieval from storage.

In a classic paper, Atkinson and Shiffrin (1968) describe the process of encoding, or transfer, of information from 'short-term' memory into the long-term memory store. Fig. 9.3 illustrates this model of memory. Attention is considered to be the gateway by which new information enters working memory, and thus the wider cognitive system. It is therefore essential to attend to new information in order to form a memory of it. As discussed in the section on attention rehabilitation, external factors can affect our ability to attend; for example, a busy or noisy environment can be highly distracting. Therefore, the

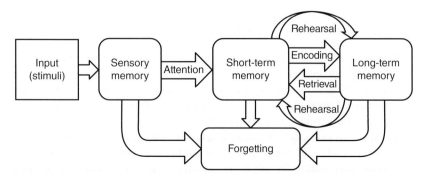

FIGURE 9.3   Memory model according to Atkinson and Shiffrin. Based on Atkinson, R.C., Shiffrin, R.M., 1968. Human memory: a proposed system and its control processes. Psychol. Learn. Motiv. 2, 89–195.

environment is also extremely important in the context of memory rehabilitation, as it can either help or hinder the process of memory formation.

The concept of 'short-term' memory was later developed and expanded upon into 'working memory' (Baddeley and Hitch, 1974). Arguing that the above model portrayed short-term memory in a simplified unitary fashion, which could only 'hold' information (rather than process and manipulate), Baddeley and Hitch suggested that working memory was multimodal, involving a central executive, visuospatial sketchpad, and phonological loop. Further reading is recommended, should you wish to understand working memory in greater detail.

Returning to the Multi Store Model, Atkinson and Shiffrin (1968) suggest that information which is more meaningful, or more emotionally salient for an individual, is both more likely to be attended to and also more likely to be consolidated and encoded into memory. They also suggest that information will be more likely to be encoded and stored if the person is exposed to it on multiple occasions. These ideas, along with the concept of errorless learning (Baddeley, 1992; Baddeley and Wilson, 1994) and the use of compensation strategies/aids to improve functioning, have been highly instrumental in the development of effective approaches to rehabilitation of memory impairments.

Consider for a moment the types of memory you have used today. If working memory is impaired, what types of memory impairment may you see in function?

## Rehabilitation of memory

As in all areas of cognitive rehabilitation, the rehabilitation of memory impairment aims to restore function, where possible, or to compensate for ongoing impairments in function.

Rehabilitation begins with education, aiming to increase the person's awareness and understanding of their own memory problems, how such impairment can impact upon their day-to-day life, and what can be done to help reduce this impact.

This sequence is to be used every morning to help increase Mark's orientation. It is really important that this information is presented to him in the same way each time and that he is not allowed the opportunity to guess.

- Hi Mark, my name is _____ I am _____.
- You are currently in the Complex Rehabilitation Unit at the Walton Centre participating in therapies to help you recover from a brain injury.
- Today is: __/__/__ and it is now ___ o'clock.
- You will be having your physiotherapy session at __:__ with *name of therapist*
- Your occupational therapy session will be at __:__ with *name of therapist*
- *insert any other appointments*
- I will just update the board with that information.

FIGURE 9.4   Script example for errorless learning.

Restorative approaches to the rehabilitation of memory are most commonly used in the early phases of rehabilitation, at times when memory impairments are at their most severe; for example, when a person is in the process of emerging from a period of post-traumatic amnesia after a traumatic brain injury (Mateer, 2005). Restorative approaches (such as visual imagery and association techniques) may also be used to help people with mild memory impairment after brain injury or stroke to improve recall of specific information (Cicerone et al., 2019).

Errorless learning is an approach which aims to prevent people from providing the wrong answer or making mistakes when learning new information or new skills (Wilson et al., 2010). It is based upon the idea that people with significant memory difficulties find it very difficult to learn from mistakes, but will learn from the correct repetition of information or actions. Errorless learning has been found to reduce confabulation, which is when a person 'fills in the gaps' in their memory with inaccurate information (Sohlberg et al., 2005).

Memory rehabilitation requires a team approach, and errorless learning is a good example of how close co-operation between professionals and family members, working to support a person, greatly assists outcome in rehabilitation. Fig. 9.4 is an example of a script which can be used by all members of a team, along with the patient's family, to deliver the same information to a patient each day, following an errorless approach.

Compensatory strategies and external aids and systems are most commonly introduced to help patients to function more independently in more generalised situations. These are typically used later in the rehabilitation process; for example, with people who are returning home or returning to work after an acquired brain injury.

*Compensatory strategies for memory impairment*

Errorless learning and other 'restorative' approaches have the potential to help people to acquire specific pieces of information and specific skills, which can be extremely beneficial (e.g., when learning names, addresses, telephone numbers, or how to call somebody on a mobile phone). However, rehabilitation aims to help people to be able to function increasingly well in their day-to-day lives, which typically will include complex and changing situations, which are ill-suited to time-intensive and specific errorless learning approaches. A significant focus of research in the area of cognitive rehabilitation has therefore focussed upon the use of compensatory strategies, aids, and systems (Wilson, 1996). The evidence base indicates that compensatory approaches are the gold standard for the rehabilitation of memory difficulties (Carney, 2005; Wilson, 2005). Examples of compensatory strategies include: use of wall-planners and prospective diaries to help people to structure their time, remind them of upcoming events to attend, or actions to take; shopping lists; to-do lists; lists of names of work colleagues or students in a class; or text-message reminders of appointments. Compensatory strategies can incorporate physical equipment (memory aids), such as notebooks or wall-planners, and more recently, technology, such as mobile phones or 'digital assistants'/'smart speakers' (with software which enables people to be sent reminders, at preset times, tailored to their needs). Compensatory strategies reduce the cognitive load on the brain by relying on the external environment, including equipment, to prompt or remind the individual to do something or recall something important to them.

*Inpatient strategies*

1. Use of a whiteboard with the date visible, along with activities/appointments/scheduled sessions for the day ahead.
2. Use of alarms to set reminders for sessions and appointments.
3. Diaries, journals, mobile phone applications/reminders, timetables, post-it notes.
4. Ensuring an organised and tidy environment.

*Community strategies*

1. Setting an alarm/timer on the oven or in the kitchen to support with cooking.
2. Writing down step-by-step instructions to complete a task, and keeping the instructions visible and close to where the task is to be done.
3. Using a prospective diary to plan appointments, as well as other activities.
4. Using a calendar which is visible on the wall.
5. Having a set place to keep belongings, such as keys and mobile phone.
6. Having a note pad next to the telephone.
7. Labelling cupboards.
8. Setting up automated reminders to be delivered to a person's mobile phone to remind them of things to do. Examples could include:
    i. Appointments to attend
    ii. When to take medications
    iii. When to go to the shops (and a list of what to buy)
    iv. When to take a moment to rest or relax
    v. Reminders to call a friend or to meet a friend for lunch.
    vi. Reminders to put the bins outside, or to take them back in.

Such reminders are useful but work best when varied, so that they do not become just 'background noise'. They also work best if they can be 'snoozed' but not dismissed until they have been acted upon.

## Case study: Isha

A female within a hospital setting has significant cognitive impairment. She is inconsistently orientated, struggles to recall the correct date and year, sometimes believes she has been at school or home, and is unable to recall the reason why she is in hospital. She is having difficulties recalling events from the last 15 years, therefore sometimes the details of past events get mixed up, and what is recalled is an amalgamation of events occurring at different times in her life. Sometimes she confabulates based on cues in her environment, recent conversation or what she has seen on the news. As she is struggling to self-monitor and detect errors in performance, she is being corrected repeatedly which is causing frustration and embarrassment.

1. What types of memory have been affected for Isha?
2. How may you assess her memory in more detail?
3. What cognitive rehabilitation approaches could be used to best support Isha?

## Case study: Philip

A young male within the community, who attends college, plays badminton, and has a busy social life, sustained a mild traumatic brain injury 1 year ago. He is missing important meetings and is turning up at the wrong time for matches.

1. What aspects of Philip's memory have been affected?
2. Which strategies could you introduce to support Philip in the community?

# Perception

Perception is the process of organising, integrating, interpreting, and representing information received from our senses (Willson et al., 2017). It is a highly automated process, which happens outside of our conscious awareness, requiring the coordinated use of our sensory organs, nervous system, dedicated perceptual centres within the brain, and also higher-order processing systems. Together, this group of connected systems interprets information flowing into our senses, and integrates it with previously obtained knowledge about the world around us, along with our, often unconscious, expectations of what will or should happen next. Perception is shaped by our lived experience of the world (our learning, memory, attention, expectations, and knowledge). Neurological illness or injury, to both the direct or indirect parts of the brain involved in perception, can have a significant effect on a person's ability to function in their day-to-day lives.

In order to assess perception, and thus inform IDT rehabilitation goals, it is helpful to consider the following theoretical subdivisions of perception. Basic visual perception can be divided into object perception (what things are) and spatial perception (where things are, relative to the individual).

*Object perception*
Object perception comprises:

1. The ability to identify and perceive the boundaries of objects
2. The ability to perceive areas of light and darkness
3. The ability to perceive colours
4. The ability to discriminate objects from their background, and to discriminate overlapping objects, for example, identifying a white T-shirt lying on a white bedsheet
5. The ability to perceive the relative size of an object
6. The ability to recognise an object's function/nature
7. The ability to name an object

Difficulties with object perception are called visual agnosia. Visual agnosia is subclassified into 'apperceptive visual agnosia' and 'associative visual agnosia' (Humphreys and Riddoch, 1987). Apperceptive visual agnosia is an impairment with forming a whole percept of an object from its component visual parts, arising from damage to areas of the brain's cortex responsible for the more fundamental elements of visual perception listed above (Warrington and James, 1988). Associative agnosia is in impairment with the identification of an object, despite being able to perceive its component parts (Rubens and Benson, 1971). Associative agnosia is distinct from anomia, the inability to recall an object's name, despite being able to identify its function or nature.

The earlier stages of object perception occur close to the poles of the occipital lobe, generally radiating outwards with increasing complexity. Object identification and naming occurs in the ventral regions of the temporal lobes, adjacent to and continuing from the fundamental visual perception centres in the occipital lobes (Milner and Goodale, 1995).

*Spatial perception*
Spatial perception consists of the ability to locate an object in space to indicate how far and in which direction it is from the viewer. Spatial perception occurs in the ventral region of the occipital lobes, on the boundary of the parietal lobes and primarily within the parietal lobes.

The control and direction of perception around 'the visual and perceptual space' surrounding a person is directed by the frontal lobes. Therefore damage, disconnection, or disruption to regions of the frontal lobes, and their connections to the parietal lobes, can result in 'spatial inattention' or in visual neglect. This is a failure to be aware of information from either the left or the right side of the person's subjective perceptual environment or of their own body, and can result in problems such as only eating from one half of the plate, only brushing one side of teeth or hair, or an inability to 'see' one side of their visual space, despite the fundamental visual perception pathways being intact (Halligan et al., 2003).

# Rehabilitation of cognitive–perceptual impairment

Identification and explanation of the specific nature of cognitive–perceptual impairment is key to enabling patients to understand and adapt to their perceptual difficulties. The use of compensatory systems is also recommended, including modification of the person's environment and also assistance to use less-impaired sensory modalities to partially compensate for perceptual difficulties in a particular sensory pathway.

Examples of rehabilitation strategies may include:

1. Education of deficits to increase the person's awareness and to support self-management.
2. Visual object perception; encourage the person to organise their environment, such as keeping things in the same place, using labels, and colour coding. Transferring certain material, such as shampoo and shower gel, into highly distinctive and consistent containers, to highlight objects that are difficult to identify or to distinguish.
3. Spatial inattention/unilateral neglect; when working with a person with spatial neglect, it is recommended to approach and stand on their nonaffected side, and gradually, as sessions progress, to work towards standing more central, to increase awareness of their midline.
4. Encouraging people to hold books at an angle of 45°, or greater, to reduce the effects of left- or right-sided neglect. Encouraging people to place their hand or an object, such as a bookmark, at the neglected side of the page and to practice 'reading up to it' (Zihl, 2010).

# Apraxia

Apraxia is an impairment of intentional, skilled, or practiced action. Apraxia is often divided into the following subtypes:

1. 'Ideational apraxia' is an impaired concept of action-oriented behaviour (Baxter and Warrington, 1986). People with ideational apraxia may misuse objects or carry out actions in the wrong sequence. For example, attempting to put a comb in the mouth rather than a toothbrush.
2. 'Ideomotor apraxia' is an impaired execution of the planned movement of a task (Heilman et al., 1982). This includes issues with direction, timing, and force of movement, which are unrelated to any physical impairment. For example, unintentionally banging a cup of tea down on the table, or shaving using a side-to-side motion, rather than an up-and-down motion.

*Rehabilitation of apraxia*
There is most evidence in favour of strategy training approaches to the rehabilitation to apraxia. Strategy training focusses upon the promotion of generalisable skills through self-monitoring and correction of action (Worthington, 2016).

An 'errorless learning' approach, as discussed in the section above with regard to memory rehabilitation, can be used to promote successful action. For example, a patient could be presented with only the items required for brushing their teeth, rather than their whole wash bag at once. An errorless learning approach would begin by directing the person to each of the items in sequence. Over time, support would be gradually reduced, such that the person is required to select an increasing number of washbag items themselves, beginning with the final item to be used and working backwards. In addition, simplifying and grading the complexity of the task can help. Educating the person about their difficulties, and giving feedback on their performance, can also be beneficial.

## Cognitive fatigue

Fatigue is one of the most commonly reported problems after acquired brain injury. Fatigue following brain injury is often referred to as cognitive or 'central' fatigue, whereby people can feel intensely fatigued irrespective of their physical energy expenditure (Belmont et al., 2006). It is important to remember that, in all of us, our brains account for around 20% of our entire energy expenditure. It is very possible that, after an acquired brain injury, the brain is working harder than before to try to accomplish tasks.

Cognitive fatigue is often reported to be the most debilitating consequence of brain injury, having an impact on all areas of life (Malley, 2014). As the pace of modern life is fast, and prior to a brain injury people live fast-paced lifestyles, adapting to cognitive fatigue can be a huge challenge. In rehabilitation we often see a 'boom and bust' pattern of behaviour, whereby patients report doing lots when they feel well and energised, only to hit a wall and collapse when energy has been expended.

Take a moment to think about what you consider to be rest and stimulation? Is watching a programme on TV always restful?

Rest and stimulation following brain injury, compared to preinjury 'rest' and 'stimulation', are extremely different. Postinjury rest means reducing or extinguishing all cognitive demands, for example, turning the TV and radio off and diming the lights. The level of postinjury stimulation that a patient is able to tolerate may have changed drastically; for example, a 5-minute conversation might be all the person can endure before experiencing fatigue.

Cognitive fatigue might present in different ways, for example, difficulties in processing information, reduced attention, disturbed sleep, struggling to initiate and make decisions, low mood, and increased anxiety. Fatigue can sometimes be mistaken for poor motivation, or 'being lazy', therefore education for partners and other family members is key.

Take a moment to think about the last time you were tired, how motivated were you?

Over stimulation can have a significant impact on levels of cognitive fatigue which can then affect cognitive function in general, thus limiting functional ability/engagement. It is therefore important to consider, with the IDT, the amount of stimulation a patient is subject to over a 24-hour period, and how levels of stimulation can vary over the course of a day.

## Management of fatigue

1. As a team, it is important to find the balance between rest and stimulating activities. Teams must discuss and share timetables and therapeutic activities, and work collaboratively when fatigue is a factor that impacts engagement and success.
2. Provide education on fatigue, normalise cognitive fatigue following injury/illness, and discuss the boom and bust pattern which is so often observed.
3. Where possible, have the person identify their fatigue early warning signs and triggers. Keeping a fatigue diary with rating scales can be helpful to identify patterns.
4. Discuss quality versus quantity, not pushing too hard or setting unrealistic expectations, and spacing out goals over time.
5. Discuss how to take rest breaks during tasks.
6. Discuss how to take regular rest breaks during the day.
7. During rest breaks make sure that it is restful, as little background noise as possible and minimal interruptions.
8. Explore relaxation/mindfulness as a way of remaining in the present moment and allowing the mind to switch off.

## Executive functions

Executive functioning is the 'highest' level of cognitive functioning (Cicerone and Giancino, 1992) referred to as a 'complex set of supervisory functions that are involved in the control of mental processes' (Spikman et al., 2017 in Wilson et al., 2017). Executive functioning refers to the abilities required to organise and direct other cognitive skills towards achieving a specific desired goal. Collaboratively, they enable people to adapt to new and novel situations, whereas situations which are familiar and predictable place much less demand upon the brain (and thus executive functions). Executive functions therefore allow people to get by in the real world and to pursue goals that are meaningful to them (Burgess and Simons, 2005). Executive functions collectively are often referred to as the 'managing director' of the brain, or the 'conductor' of the brain's orchestra; they play a vital role in coordinating and overseeing the many other cognitive processes described above, and enable them to take appropriate action in an integrated manner (Goldberg, 2009; Maskill and Tempest, 2017).

Ylvisaker and Szerekeres (1989) propose that executive function is comprised of eight key elements:

1. Goal-setting
2. Planning
3. Problem solving
4. Organisation
5. Self-initiation
6. Self-direction
7. Self-inhibition
8. Self-monitoring/self-correction

There is evidence that many interrelated parts of the brain are involved in executive functioning. However, the prefrontal cortex of the frontal lobes is generally considered to be essential to the successful operation of these higher-order skills. Baddley and Wilson (1988) introduced the term dysexecutive syndrome to describe people who have significant difficulties with executive functioning. The 'dysexecutive syndrome' lies at the extreme end of the spectrum of impairment of executive functioning, characterised by impulsivity, disinhibition, difficulty considering the consequences of actions, difficulty considering the viewpoints of others and changes in personality associated with the above. However, impaired executive functioning can also present as the opposite of this syndrome; rather than becoming more impulsive, a person can have difficulty initiating action and become very passive.

All impairments of executive functioning tend to make it more difficult for people to organise, initiate, control, or stop their behaviour, in order to achieve a desired goal. Executive dysfunction has therefore been termed 'goal neglect' (Duncan et al., 1995), which can be a useful, simplified, way of conceptualising and explaining executive impairment.

## Executive function in daily life

Executive or higher-order skills are critical for our successful functioning in various societal roles, including self-care and home management, leisure and social activities, and in work or education. These roles all place a set of cognitive demands upon us, which require us to deal with novel and changing circumstances and adapt our behaviour accordingly (Burgess and Simons, 2005; Maskill and Tempest, 2017). Maskill and Tempest (2017) propose a categorisation of executive function into four broad areas of skills required for the performance of activities of daily living.

These areas are:

1. Initiation and termination elements of a task.
2. Goal setting.
3. Planning and organisation.
4. Adaptation and flexibility.

Some examples of activities and tasks requiring executive function are listed below, but this is by no means an exhaustive list, as executive skills will depend on an individual's roles, responsibilities, and interests.

1. Preparing a meal.
2. Finding a route to somewhere you have not been before.
3. Following new and novel instructions (e.g., putting flat pack furniture together).
4. Solving a problem/dealing with an unforeseen issue (e.g., what to do if a household appliance breaks down).
5. Planning ahead, balancing your commitments across your day, week, month, and year ahead.
6. Pulling together a presentation or completing a job application.
7. Household management (e.g., managing shopping, cleaning, laundry, and home maintenance).
8. Childcare/parenting.
9. Planning a holiday.
10. Planning and organising a new kitchen.
11. Work and education skills.

Considering that the tasks highlighted above are only a small portion of those that make up our busy modern lives, we can recognise that balancing such skills can be a challenge for us all, even with intact executive skills. For people with executive dysfunction, however, the challenge of managing the competing demands of daily living is magnified. Dependent on how their cognitive difficulties present, the individual may struggle with organisation, planning, or time management, and if insight is impaired, they may not even recognise or be aware of their difficulties, and so may not be motivated to work to change their situation.

*How executive dysfunction may present*
Difficulties with executive functioning may present subtly and may not be obvious to another person in general conversation. However, as illustrated above, such difficulties can be devastating to an individual's quality of life. Such difficulties may present as a subtle feeling that something is just not 'right', or family members may describe a change in their loved one's personality, sense of humor, or ability to 'get on' with other people. The nature of an individual's environment may mask the severity of executive dysfunction. For example, inpatient and residential settings are very structured in nature, meals are brought to patients or residents at set times, therapists come to collect people from their rooms for treatment sessions, and family or staff do their washing and shopping for them. The support provided in such situations may mean that difficulties with self-directed action are not hugely apparent, as minimal day-to-day demands are placed upon the patient or resident. Whilst the structure of such environments helps to support people with executive difficulties, it also means their problems can be masked and that the extent of the difficulties may only become apparent

once they are discharged home. If the difficulties have not been highlighted before, this can mean that people do not receive the help and support they need for community living. This can be particularly evident for patients who have no discernible physical deficits and who may be very coherent in communication. If members of staff do not have the time or experience in assessing such seemingly subtle difficulties, such patients can miss out on appropriate support in the early stages of rehabilitation. Further reading on the 'frontal lobe paradox' (Walsh, 1985) is recommended, specifically in relation to mental capacity (George and Gilbert, 2018).

In the community, however, executive difficulties can become more obvious as the person has much more responsibility for managing a variety of life areas dependent on their previous occupational roles (parenting, education and work, household management, and hobbies, leisure, and social engagement). The lack of enforced structure in the community means it is now the individual's responsibility to plan, organise, and structure their own time and to deal with novel problems as they spontaneously arise, all of which will now be extremely challenging for a person with impaired executive functioning.

Occupational therapists are highly skilled in supporting individuals to maximise their independence in all activities of daily living and will work with clinical neuropsychologists or clinical psychologists, who can provide more specific advice on individual presentations. Some examples of how people with executive dysfunction may present are outlined below. It is important, however, to consider other possible factors which may contribute to this presentation, including other cognitive difficulties (e.g., memory or attention), anxiety or low mood, premorbid or organic personality traits, fear, pain, fatigue or cultural issues/differences.

Below is a list of the potential ways executive dysfunction following injury/illness may present:

1. Impaired Insight/self-awareness
2. Inability to set realistic goals
3. Rigidity/difficulty accepting or adapting to the effects of illness/injury
4. Issues with relating to others (social cognition)
5. Poor self-care
6. Apparent low motivation (self-initiation issues)
7. Issues with behaviour/compliance
8. Poor 'follow-through' with tasks/poor progress
9. Inconsistency
10. Issues with recalling information
11. Problems with organisation
12. Difficult to 'keep on track', in tasks or in conversation.
13. Disinhibition (impulsivity), for example, excessive talking, eating, smoking, spending money, hoarding, etc.

## Case study: Anne

Anne is in her early 60s. Her family is concerned about some subtle but ongoing changes following her brain haemorrhage. They report she comes across as a little 'odd' now, in that she seems to wander around the ward and takes a lot of interest in what is going on with other patients, sometimes interrupting their conversations with relatives. They find this very embarrassing, as she was always very polite and well mannered. They report Anne was always an 'elegant lady', but that she no longer appears to attend to her appearance quite the same. The catering staff has noticed that at meal times she tends to 'wolf down' her food and her table manners do not seem to 'fit' with what Anne would have been like previously.

## Case study: Rashid

Rashid is making a good physical recovery from his traumatic brain injury. He is in his second year at university and is keen to maintain links with the university in the hope that he will soon be able to return to his course. However, through discussion, although maintaining his place at university is his key focus, he is not keeping on top of the basic level of communication with the university, he is not responding to emails, and has not returned the university administration calls. His parents have offered to help with this, but he is insistent he can manage. It also becomes apparent that he has not been keeping a check on his personal finances and has not been dealing with his landlord.

## Reflective questions

Take a moment to consider the following:

- Have you encountered patients with similar difficulties?
- Considering your learning so far, what executive difficulties do you think these patients could be experiencing?
- How may you assess executive functioning in more detail?
- What may be your role when working with the above two patients?
- What may be the barriers to engagement/successful rehabilitation?

# Rehabilitation of executive dysfunction

Interdisciplinary working is key to optimising the recovery and management of executive functioning difficulties. The treatment and management of executive dysfunction largely consists of approaches aimed at restoring the specific skill affected, teaching the individual strategies to compensate for their difficulties, and putting in place adaptive measures for their ongoing difficulties (Chung et al., 2013; Cicerone and Giacino, 1992). Evidence exists for the success of strategy training to address planning and problem-solving issues, and for improving self-awareness through providing feedback (Tate et al., 2014). In clinical practice, the approach must be tailored to the person's specific goals and should be developed collaboratively with the patient, to ensure they use systems that are relevant to them, often those they may have relied upon preinjury. If the patient presents with poor self-awareness, this should be addressed as a priority to help them to be able to monitor their own performance (self-monitoring is a key executive skill). By educating patients about their executive difficulties and how the frontal lobes function, increased self-awareness may help them to take more responsibility, so they can self-manage their difficulties. Some examples of strategies and interventions are listed below; however, this is by no means an exhaustive list.

1. Prompt sheets, alarms, visual cues as reminders.
2. Practice of relevant daily activities using a graded approach. Grading can involve task complexity, amount/type of cuing/prompting/assistance given. This can be across a wide array of daily tasks relevant to the person.
3. Problem-solving tasks.
4. Multiple errands tests.
5. Goal setting.
6. Prediction/evaluation of task.
7. Feedback including self-reflection, verbal feedback from staff and video feedback.
8. Apps for phone, tablets, other technology.

## Summary

This chapter has hopefully offered a straightforward introduction to the topic of cognition, aimed at all members of an IDT, by providing an overview of attention, memory, perception, apraxia, cognitive fatigue, and executive function. We have provided an explanation of each cognitive skill and illustrated how cognitive impairments may manifest clinically. Examples of how cognitive problems may affect patients across a variety of rehabilitation settings has been discussed, and we have asked the reader throughout, to reflect on and consider their own personal practice and how they can support patients with cognitive impairment. We have highlighted the importance of a 24-hour approach to the management and rehabilitation of cognitive problems, and emphasised the importance of an interdisciplinary approach. We now challenge the reader to take their learning forward and consider what they can do to support patients with cognitive difficulties to ultimately optimise successful rehabilitation outcomes.

## References

Atkinson, R.C., Shiffrin, R.M., 1968. Human memory: a proposed system and its control processes. Psychol. Learn. Motiv. 2, 89–195.

Baddeley, A., 1992. Implicit memory and errorless learning: a link between cognitive theory and neuropsychological rehabilitation? In: Squire, L.R., Butters, N. (Eds.), Neuropsychology of Memory, second ed. The Guilford Press, New York.

Baddeley, A., Hitch, G., 1974. Working memory. Psychol. Learn. Motiv. 8, 47–89.

Baddeley, A., Wilson, B., 1988. Frontal amnesia and the dysexecutive syndrome. Brain Cognit. 7 (2), 212–230.

Baxter, D.M., Warrington, E.K., 1986. Ideational agraphia: a single case study. J. Neurol. Neurosurg. Psychiatry 49 (4), 369–374.

Belmont, A., Agar, N., Hugeron, C., Gallais, B., Azouvi, P., 2006. Fatigue and traumatic brain injury. Ann. Readapt. Med. Phys. 49, 370–374.

Ben-Yishay, Y., Diller, L., 2008. Kurt Goldstein's holistic ideas—an alternative, or complementary, approach to the management of traumatically brain-injured individuals. US Neurol. 04 (01), 79.

Burgess, P.W. and Simons, J.S. (2005). Theories of frontal lobe executive function: clinical applications. In: P.W. Halligan and D.T. Wade (Eds.), Effectiveness of Rehabilitation for Cognitive Deficits. New York: Oxford University Press; pp. 211–212

Carney, N., 2005. Cognitive rehabilitation outcomes for traumatic brain injury. The effective treatment of memory-related disabilities. In: Halligan, P., Wade, D.T. (Eds.), The Effectiveness of Rehabilitation for Cognitive Deficits. Oxford University Press, London, pp. 295–318.

Casaletto, K.B., Heaton, R.K., 2017. Neuropsychological assessment: past and future. J. Int. Neuropsychol. Soc. 23 (9-10), 778–790.

Chung, C.S., Pollock, A., et al., 2013. Cognitive rehabilitation for executive dysfunction in adults with stroke or other adult non-progressive acquired brain damage. Cochrane Database Syst. Rev. 4, Cd008391.

Cicerone, K., Giacino, J.T., 1992. Remediation of executive function deficits after traumatic brain injury. NeuroRehabilitation 2 (3), 12–22.

Cicerone, K., Goldin, Y., Ganci, K., Rosenbaum, A., Wethe, J., Langenbahn, D., Malec, J., Bergquist, T., Kingsley, K., Nagele, D., Trexler, L., Fraas, M., Bogdanova, Y., Harley, J., 2019. Evidence-based cognitive rehabilitation: systematic review of the literature from 2009 through 2014. Arch. Phys. Med. Rehab. 100. doi:10.1016/j.apmr.2019.02.011.

Craik, F.I.M., Lockhart, R.S., 1972. Levels of processing: a framework for memory research. J. Learn. Verbal Behav. 1, 671–684.

C.M. van Heugten Spikman, J.M., Krasny-Pacini, A., Limond, J., Chevignard, M., 2017. Rehabilitation of executive functions. In: Wilson, B.A., Winegardner, J., Ownsworth, T. (Eds.), Neuropsychological Rehabilitation. Routledge, London, pp. 172–178.

C.M. van Heugten Wilson, B.A, Mole, J., Manly, T., 2017. Rehabilitation of attention disorder. In: Wilson, B.A., Winegardner, J., Ownsworth, T. (Eds.), Neuropsychological Rehabilitation Routledge, London.

Duncan, J., 2013. The structure of cognition: attentional episodes in mind and brain. Neuron 80 (1), 35–50. doi:10.1016/j.neuron.2013.09.015.

Worthington, A., 2016. Treatments and technologies in the rehabilitation of apraxia and action disorganisation syndrome: a review. Neurorehabilitation 39 (1), 163–174.

Duncan, J., Burgess, P., Emslie, H., 1995. Fluid intelligence after frontal lobe lesions. Neuropsychologia 33 (3), 261–268.

George, M.S., Gilbert, S., 2018. Mental Capacity Act (2005) assessments: why everyone needs to know about the frontal lobe paradox. Neuropsychologist 5, 59–66.

Goldberg, E., 2009. The New Executive Brain: Frontal Lobes in a Complex World. Oxford Unversty Press, New York.

Goshke, K., 1996. Rembering what to do: explicit and implicit memory for intentions. In: Einstein, G.O., Brandimonte, M.A. (Eds.), Prospective Memory: Theory and Applications. Psychology Press, New York, pp. 53–59.

Halligan, P.W., Fink, G.R., Marshall, J.C., Vallar, G., 2003. Spatial cognition: evidence from visual neglect. Trends Cogn. Sci. 7 (3), 125–133. doi:10.1016/S1364-6613(03)00032-9.

Heilman, K.M., Rothi, L.J., Valenstein, E., 1982. Two forms of ideomotor apraxia. Neurology 32 (4), 342–346.

Hollingworth, H.L., 1913. Characteristic differences between recall and recognition. Am. J. Psychol. 24 (4), 532–544.

Humphreys, G.W., Riddoch, M.J., 1987. The fractionation of visual agnosia. In: Humphreys, G.W., Riddoch, M.J. (Eds.), In:Visual Object Processing: A Cognitive Neuropsychological Approach. Routledge, pp. 281–306.

Kinsella, G.J., 1998. Assessment of attention following traumatic brain injury: a review. Neuropsychol. Rehab. 8 (3), 351–375. doi:10.1080/713755576.

Malia, K., 1997. Insight after brain injury: what does it mean? J. Cogn. Rehab. 15 (3), 10–16.

Malley, D., Gracey, F., Wheatcroft, J., 2014. Fatigue After Acquired Brain Injury a Model to Guide Clinical Management. Advances in Clinical Neuroscience & Rehabilitation. ACNR, Vol. 14, pp. 17–19.

Maskill, L., Tempest, S., 2017. Neuropsychology for Occupational Therapists. Cognition in Occupational Performance, fourth ed. Wiley, Oxford, p. 165.

Mateer, C.A., 2005. Fundamentals of cognitive rehabilitation. In: Halligan, P.W., Wade, D.T (Eds.), Effectiveness of Rehabilitation for Cognitive Deficits. Oxford University Press, London, pp. 21–31.

Milner, D.A., Goodale, M.A., 1995. The Visual Brain in Action. Oxford University Press, London.

Nadel, L., Moscovitch, M., 1997. Memory consolidation, retrograde amnesia and the hippocampal complex. Curr. Opin. Neurobiol. 7 (2), 217–227.

Rubens, A.B., Benson, F., 1971. Associate visual agnosia. Arch. Neurol. 24 (4), 305–316.

Schkade, J., Schultz, S., 1992. Occupational adaptation: toward a holistic approach for contemporary practice, part 1. Am. J. Occup. Ther. 46 (9), 829–837.

Sohlberg, M.M., Ehlhardt, L., Kennedy, M., 2005. Instructional techniques in cognitive rehabilitation: a preliminary report. Semin. Speech Lang. 26 (4), 268–279.

Sohlberg, M.M., Mateer, C.A., 2001. Cognitive Rehabilitation: An Integrative Neuropsychological Approach. Guilford Press, New York.

Sperling, G.,1960. The information available in brief visual presentations. Psychological monographs: general and applied, 74 (11), 1.

Squire, L.R., Zola, S.M., 1998. Episodic memory, semantic memory and amnesia. Hippocampus 8 (3), 205–211.

Tate, R., Kennedy, M., Ponsford, J., Dougla., J., Velikonja, D., Bayley, M., Stergiou-Kita, M., 2014. INCOG recommendations for management of cognition following traumatic brain injury, part III: executive function and self-awareness. J. Head Trauma Rehab. 29 (4), 338–352. doi:10.1097/HTR.0000000000000068.

Tulving, E., 1972. Episodic and semantic memory. In: Tulving, E., Donaldson, W. (Eds.), Organization of Memory. Academic Press, New York, pp. 381–402.

Van Heugten, C.M. Fish, J., 2017. Rehabilitation of attention disorder. In: Wilson, B.A., Winegardner, J., Ownsworth, T. (Eds.), Neuropsychological Rehabilitation: The International Handbook. Routledge, Oxford, pp. 172–178.

Walsh, K.W., 1985. Understanding Brain Damage: A Primer of Neuropsychological Evaluation. Longman Group Ltd, London.

Warrington, E.K., James, M., 1988. Visual apperceptive agnosia: a clinico-anatomical study of three cases. In: Davidoff, J.B. (Ed.), Brain and Behaviour: Critical Concepts in Psychology, vol. 1. Routledge, London, pp. 361–381.

Wilson, B.A., 1996. A Practical Framework for understanding compensatory behaviour in people with organic memory impairment. Memory 4 (5), 465–486.

Wilson, B.A., 2005. The effective treatment of memory-related disabilities. In: Halligan, P., Wade, D.T. (Eds.), The Effectiveness of Rehabilitation for Cognitive Deficits. Oxford University Press, London, pp. 143–154.

Wilson, B.A., Baddeley, A.D., Evans, J., Shiel, A., 1994. Errorless learning in the rehabilitation of memory impaired people. Neuropsychol. Rehab. 4, 307–326.

Wilson, B.A., Baddeley, A., Evans, J., Shiel, A., 2010. Errorless learning in the rehabilitation of memory impaired people. Neuropsychol. Rehab. 4 (3), 307–326.

Ylvisaker, M., Szekeres, S.F., 1989. Metacognitive and executive impairments in head-injured children and adults. Topics in Language Disorders. 9 (2), 34–49. https://doi.org/10.1097/00011363-198903000-00005.

Zihl, J., 2010. Rehabilitation of Visual Disorders of Brain Injury. Psychology Press, London.

Chapter 10

# Communication disorders in rehabilitation: an interdisciplinary approach

Elaine Bailey and Lisa Barklin

## Chapter outline

## Abstract

A communication disorder is described as any disorder that affects an individual's ability to comprehend, detect, or apply language and speech in order to engage in discourse effectively with others (Jumonville, 2012). Even the simplest form of communication requires numerous complex processes to take place. A breakdown can occur in any of those processes, and can result in a wide range of life-changing symptoms. Some

A Practical Approach to Interdisciplinary Complex Rehabilitation.
DOI: https://doi.org/10.1016/B978-0-7020-8276-4.00010-2

of these symptoms may include an inability to produce intelligible speech, difficulty understanding ones' own language, suddenly being unable to read or write, or maybe a combination of all of these symptoms. Tasks previously taken for granted become challenging—imagine not being able to ask a loved one how their day was, not being able to read or send a simple text, write a shopping list, or convey important decisions about your own life. Patients with communication difficulties are vulnerable, and at risk of decisions being made for them about their future. This results in decisions about health care and discharges being made, that do not reflect the patient's choice. Engaging in a holistic approach and working collaboratively with the interdisciplinary team is fundamental to ensuring that a person with communication difficulties is able to make informed choices and participate fully in the decision-making process.

**Keywords**
Communication disorders; Rehabilitation and wellbeing; Interdisciplinary working; Mental capacity assessment; Informed choice; Alternative and augmentative communication; Assistive technology

## Aim

The aim of this chapter is to discuss the impact of communication on the rehabilitation journey and the positive influence that interdisciplinary team working has on a patient's outcome.

## Overview

This chapter will discuss communication disorders and their impact on a person's wellbeing and rehabilitation journey. The role of the speech and language therapist (SLT) will be discussed, and we will analyse how the interdisciplinary team (IDT) contributes to the rehabilitation process of communication disorders.

## Definition of communication

Communication is the process of sending and receiving messages through verbal and nonverbal means. Communication is said to be 'the creation and exchange of meaning' (Nordguist, 2019).
    Communication involves:

1. Exchange of information
2. Intent
3. Meaning
4. Interpretation

## Role of speech and language therapists

1. Assess, diagnose, and manage communication difficulties.
2. To find a functional means of communication, enabling patients to express themselves in the most effective way.

3. Direct or indirect intervention (or a combination of both).
4. Work closely with other members of the IDT.
5. Are involved in ensuring capacity assessments and information are provided in the most accessible way.
6. Support families and carers to communicate effectively with their loved one.

## The communication cycle

Take a simple, everyday question and response:

How are you today? I'm fine thank you.

This is a common exchange that can be heard to take place between individuals in numerous different settings and environments. The exchange may take place face to face in close proximity, or there may be distance involved, with the exchange being shouted across a street, over the telephone, etc. Although it seems like a simple exchange, many processes need to take place in order for this everyday communication to be effective.

The listener needs to be able to hear the words and understand the language as being familiar to them. The words and intonation need to be interpreted as a question. The tense needs to be understood (*are* rather than *were*), as does the pronoun (*you* as opposed to *they/he/she*).

The response requires some thought—Do I want to answer the question? Do I want to answer truthfully? Am I going to answer truthfully? The type of response will be dependent on the relationship between the two communicators. An unconscious internal dialogue takes place regarding the most appropriate way to answer the question. For example, the response to an acquaintance, or a manager (I'm fine thanks), may be different to the response to a close friend (I'm not great, I've had a bad morning, I locked myself out of my house and missed my bus).

In order to give the response, the respondent needs to access their word store and select the correct words to convey the required person (I), tense (am, was), word order (I'm fine thank you, not fine I'm you thank) and intonation (a statement vs. a question). The brain then needs to activate the correct breathing pattern and the vocal cords in order for vocalisation to take place. Coordination of the lips and tongue takes place to ensure that the correct sounds are articulated, in the correct order, and to ensure the utterance is audible, intelligible, and without error. This all happens in a matter of milliseconds.

The response then needs to be interpreted by the conversation partner. This often takes place in a busy, noisy environment, with other conversations taking place, whilst thinking about other priorities simultaneously.

So even the simplest form of communication requires numerous complex processes to take place. Given the complexity of communication following injury to the brain, a breakdown can occur in any of the above steps, resulting in a communication disorder.

## The impact of communication disorders

What would life be like if you couldn't communicate?

Imagine being unable to send a quick text to say that you will be home late, not having the language ability to explain how you are feeling, and not being able to ask your children what they did at school today.

Most of our happiness and sadness comes from our interactions with others, whether directly or indirectly, and how we perceive such interactions determines the quality of our life experiences (Code, 2003). Depression is frequently experienced by both the person with communication difficulties and those close to them (Code, 2003).

Impact on the person with communication difficulties:

1. Change in own identity
2. Role within relationships
3. Interactions deteriorate
4. Social interaction and participation reduces
5. Decline in confidence
6. Depression and other mental health issues

Impact on the family and carers:

1. High levels of anxiety
2. Feeling trapped and isolated

## Definition of a communication disorder

A communication disorder is described as any disorder that affects an individual's ability to comprehend, detect, or apply language and speech to engage in discourse effectively with others (Jumonville, 2012). The delays and disorders can range from simple sound substitution to the inability to understand or use one's native language (Gleason, 2001).

Broca's and Wernicke's aphasia are terms that are sometimes discussed in relation to brain function and language (Fig. 10.1). They may be used to label a patient's communication difficulty, with Broca's aphasia describing expressive aphasia, and Wernicke's aphasia describing receptive aphasia.

However, *communication difficulties are rarely this distinct*. From an SLT's perspective, it is important to describe the communication difficulty as a whole, and establish the level of impairment and functional impact, rather than establishing the 'label'.

SLTs carry out assessments that enable them to describe the presenting communication problem and establish the level of impairment and functional impact. An intervention programme can then be devised in order to target the specific area of breakdown and allow a means of functional communication to be investigated and developed.

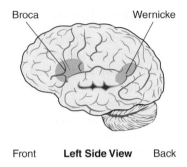

FIGURE 10.1    Location of Broca's and Wernicke's areas. From National Institute on Deafness and Other Communication Disorders (NIDCD), 2010. Available at: https://www.nidcd.nih.gov/health/aphasia. Accessed October 7, 2021.

## Types of communication disorders

### Dysphasia

In the majority of the population, where a person is right handed, language is controlled by the dominant left cerebral hemisphere. A left-sided brain insult will frequently result in acquired language difficulties. An acquired language disorder is known as aphasia, also called dysphasia. The two words aphasia and dysphasia are often used interchangeably, although it should be noted that some clinicians may use aphasia to describe a total loss, and dysphasia to describe a partial loss. Impairments can present in the areas of understanding verbal and written language and expressing verbal and written language.

There is a range of psycholinguistic theoretical models attempting to explain how our brains process language and how we talk/write to communicate thoughts and opinions. One of the models commonly used in practice is the psycholinguistic assessment of language processing in aphasia (Kay et al., 1996)—this is known as the PALPA. The PALPA provides a range of assessments to pinpoint breakdown in the proposed cognitive linguistic model of language comprehension and production (Fig. 10.2). The assessment provides a range of subtests that enable the area of language breakdown to be identified, meaning that the specific breakdown can then be targeted in intervention. It is not within the remit of this chapter to discuss the implementation of the PALPA in detail, further reading is required should the reader wish to familiarise themselves with the model.

### Dysarthria

Dysarthria is a condition in which the muscles used for speech are weak and there is difficulty controlling them. Dysarthria is often characterised by slurred or slow speech that can be difficult to understand.

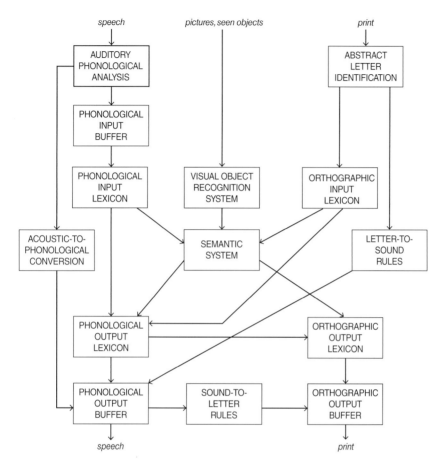

**FIGURE 10.2**   PALPA model (Kay et al., 1996). Reproduced with permission from Taylor & Francis Ltd. (www.tandfonline.com).

Signs and symptoms of dysarthria vary, depending on the underlying cause and the type of dysarthria, and may include:

1. Slurred speech
2. Slow speech
3. Inability to speak louder than a whisper or speaking too loudly
4. Rapid speech that is difficult to understand
5. Nasal, raspy, or strained voice
6. Uneven or abnormal speech rhythm
7. Uneven speech volume
8. Monotone speech
9. Difficulty moving the tongue or facial muscles

## Dyspraxia

A person with verbal dyspraxia has difficulty placing muscles in the correct position to produce speech. The muscles have not been damaged. The messages from the brain that tell the muscles what to do have been affected.

The person usually knows what they want to say, but has difficulty saying it. The wrong sounds may be articulated, or sometimes no sound at all. This can be frustrating for the speaker as a word may come out correctly one minute and incorrectly the next.

A person with dyspraxia may:

1. not be able to speak or gesture at all
2. sometimes be able to produce 'automatic' speech, such as counting, common phrases, or greetings such as 'fine, thanks', or 'OK' or swear words
3. make searching movements with their mouth and tongue, trying to find the right position for what they want to say
4. get stuck on a sound or word
5. have speech which sounds 'jumbled up' and be difficult to understand
6. have pauses and hesitations in their speech, and
7. it may take a lot of effort for them to try and speak.

## Dysphonia

Dysphonia presents as trouble voicing when trying to talk, including having no voice, hoarseness, and change in pitch or quality of voice.

## Dysfluency

Dysfluent speech is the disruption of the flow and timing of speech by repetition of sounds, syllables or words, sound prolongation, and/or blocking on sounds, silent, or audible (Bloodstein and Bernstein Ratner, 2008). Patients may experience acquired dysfluency postinjury.

## Dyslexia

Dyslexia is a difficulty that can cause problems with reading and spelling. Patients may experience acquired difficulty with reading and spelling postinjury that was not previously present.

## Dysgraphia

Dysgraphia presents as difficulty in forming letters, producing a mixture of upper/lower case letters, irregular letter sizes and shapes and unfinished letters. A person with dysgraphia will struggle to use writing as a communication tool.

## Dyscalculia

Dyscalculia is a specific difficulty in understanding numbers and numerical concepts leading to a diverse range of difficulties with mathematics, which was not present prior to injury.

## Cognitive communication disorders

Cognitive communication disorders present as difficulty with communication competence (listening, speaking, reading, writing, and conversational interaction) that result from underlying cognitive impairments (attention, memory, organisation, information processing, problem solving, and executive functions).

*Please note, patients rarely present with these symptoms in isolation and will often present with a combination of more than one of the above disorders.*

# The impact of communication disorders on the patient and their family

## Case study 1: Acquired dyslexia

Mrs. M is a 69-year-old lady who had a subarachnoid haemorrhage, hydrocephalus, and middle cerebral artery aneurysm. Premorbidly, she presented with a history of depression which she self-managed by reading novels; this allowed her to 'escape' when she was feeling low. She lives alone and was previously independent. She is a retired shop worker with six children and 16 grandchildren.

Following SLT assessment, Mrs. M was found to be following all instructions and questions appropriately. She was able to express herself in full, grammatically correct sentences and responded to complex questions and commands. She did not present with any dysarthria or dyspraxia. She presented as alert and engaged well in conversation, however, in the initial assessment it was found that Mrs. M was having difficulty recognising and reading letters. A combination of formal and informal assessments found that Mrs. M presented with difficulty identifying letters, discriminating letters, letter naming, and sounding out letters, resulting in an inability to read. She was able to write and spell without difficulty.

This impairment severely affected Mrs. M; she had previously read four to five novels a week to manage low mood, and now that she was unable to do this, the injury had a significant impact on her psychological wellbeing. She was now mistaking items in the shower, and was unable to read food labels and instructions. This in turn impacted on her independence in washing, dressing, and cooking tasks. She was unable to read texts, which impacted on her ability to keep in touch with friends and family, resulting in decreased social opportunity. She was unable to read letters and bills, which potentially would impact on her ability to return home without support. Mrs. M would wake up disorientated every morning, believing it to be Saturday. Ward staff had introduced an orientation board, but unfortunately Mrs. M could not read it, and became increasingly frustrated with the disorientation, leading to a decline in her mood. Psychological assessment found that low mood was affecting her overall cognition, in particular her ability to focus and attend to information.

SLT intervention utilised a kinesthetic feedback approach based on a technique described by Maher et al. (1998). Maher et al. (1998) discuss rehabilitation of the visual orthographic input system, in which therapy involves copying letters on to the palm of a patient's hand, thereby providing tactile as well as motor feedback. Maher et al. found that tracing letters on to their patient's hand, and with intensive intervention and practice, their patient was able to elicit word recognition via the semantic system. After 4 weeks of intensive intervention, Mrs. M displayed a significant improvement in written letter recognition. Occupational therapy repeated a shopping trip with Mrs. M, which had previously been unsuccessful and caused high levels of frustration for Mrs. M. In this second trip, Mrs. M was now able to read aisle signs, shopping lists, and food labels. The requirement for the kinesthetic feedback technique reduced, with Mrs. M being more able to recognise whole words as the intervention progressed. She quickly moved on to reading children's books, then large print novels, and read one of her favourite novels whilst on home leave. She then progressed further, to be able to read bills and appointment letters.

*Overall impact*:
The unit psychologist reported a significant increase in mood levels, which then positively impacted on cognitive function, with increased attention and ability to focus. Occupational therapies were able to engage Mrs. M in independent functional tasks, for example, personal care, shopping, and cooking. Nursing staff were able to engage with her more due to the reduced frustration she felt on the ward. She could be discharged back to living independently and could continue to manage her premorbid low mood by reading novels again.

## Case study 2: Dyscalculia

Mr. P is a 30-year-old gentleman. He was previously fit and well, living independently and working full-time. Mr. P had a right basal ganglia bleed, which resulted in physical impairment as well as moderate receptive and expressive dysphasia. He was orientated to time, place, and person and had no short-term or long-term memory issues. He was motivated for therapy and progressed well, with his communication difficulties improving to conversational level throughout his admission. However, whilst Mr. P's impairments improved in all other areas, he was found to continue to have difficulty in recognising numbers.

This residual impairment resulted in Mr. P being unable to independently manage day-to-day activities. He could not tell the time or use his bank card with his pin. He could not manage his bank account or bills; he had difficulty with budgeting and day-to-day money management. He could not recognise numbers in order to make telephone calls and could not comprehend numbers as spoken words, written words, or digits. Occupational therapists worked with Mr. P to introduce strategies to target these difficulties; a speaking clock was introduced into Mr. P's room so that he was able to know the time without having to understand the numbers. Telephone numbers were stored into his phone, meaning that Mr. P was then able to telephone friends and family independently, as he was able to read the names in his contact list. He could use contactless to pay for small purchases; however, he could not be certain that the amount he was being asked to pay was the correct amount, due to being unable to add up the total independently, or check the receipt. When paying with cash, he was unable to select the correct coins or notes, or check his change, having to rely on the shop cashier to select the correct money from an amount handed to them by Mr. P. Mr. P was therefore in a vulnerable position, and at risk of financial abuse. He was found to lack capacity around financial decisions, and following a best interest meeting, an appointee was allocated to manage his finances on his behalf. SLT intervention targeted number and money recognition, with the aim of re-establishing names for numbers, relate digits to quantities, and re-establish place value. Whilst improvement was shown, unfortunately Mr. P had not attained a level of functional recognition at the time of his discharge and was considered to be too vulnerable to live independently. He was therefore rehoused into supported living to assist with day-to-day money management, shopping, and paying bills, with a view to moving on to reduced support in the future, should his number and money recognition improve to a functional level.

## Case study 3: Cognitive communication disorder

Mr. B is a 43-year-old gentleman who was previously fit and well, living independently and working full-time. He had a fall resulting in a traumatic brain injury.

Informally Mr. B was observed to be communicating his basic needs, being able to express himself fluently, and following basic instructions and questions. He did not have any mobility issues and presented as physically well. Mr. B achieved within normal limits on all language assessments.

However, Mr. B's conversational interaction was impaired due to a cognitive communication disorder. Mr. B would talk at length about topics of his choice. He would assume that the listener had prior knowledge of a topic, including people and places. He would regularly switch topics mid conversation and provide extraneous information. This would regularly result in listener confusion and frustration for Mr. B. He did not respond to verbal or nonverbal cues from the listener; for example, if the listener stated 'I need to go now Mr. B', he would continue to talk at length to them, and would not respond to a cue such as the listener having a hand on the door, standing in the doorway ready to leave.

Mr. B's social communication was also affected, with him verbalising inappropriate comments in public, and being overfamiliar with strangers. Mr. B looked well and did not present as a person with a disability, resulting in bystanders' reduced understanding of his difficulties, and him being extremely vulnerable in the community.

The IDT worked closely with Mr. B in order to increase his awareness and insight into his communication difficulties, however his cognitive issues made it difficult for him to take the information on board and for him to carry over and generalise strategies. Work therefore focussed on providing support to his family, increasing their communication confidence and promoting positive interactions between Mr. B and his loved ones. This allowed Mr. B to have successful home leave with his family's support, and he was eventually able to be discharged home with the support of his family and a package of care.

## Supporting families

Brown et al. (2012) investigated what families needed during their loved one's rehabilitation journey, with the following key categories being identified:

1. to be included in rehabilitation
2. to be provided with hope and responsibility
3. to be able to communicate and maintain their relationship with the person with communication difficulty
4. to be given information
5. to be given support
6. to look after their own mental, emotional and physical wellbeing
7. to be able to cope with new responsibilities

These are key factors that need to be taken into account throughout the rehabilitation journey.

## IDT working

What can the whole rehabilitation team do?
   Helpful characteristics for positive interactions:

1. ability to put someone at ease
2. ability to make someone feel important
3. displaying a positive mood
4. being empathic
5. being a good communicator

These are attributes that are present across a whole IDT, and can be utilised holistically to provide the best possible environment for positive communication access. Specific strategies will be provided by the SLT based on individual patient need.

'True access means that everyone needs to be able to support communication, whenever and wherever the need arises' (Simmons-Mackie et al., 2014).

## Supporting communication for mental capacity assessments

An important role for SLTs within a rehabilitation setting is to provide support for assessing mental capacity, particularly for those patients with communication difficulties. Central to the principle of patient-centred care is the respect for an individual's right to be fully involved in decisions about all aspects of their health care. For patients with communication difficulties this can be challenging, however it is the responsibility of health care professionals to ensure that this principle is upheld.

Decision making is a complex process that involves multiple cognitive and linguistic abilities, including understanding information relevant to a decision, manipulating that information in a deliberative process, appreciating the consequences of making or not making a decision, and communicating a choice (Appelbaum and Grisso, 1988). Because capacity assessment relies heavily on language skills, demonstrating capacity is often challenging or sometimes impossible for patients with communication difficulties, and research suggests that patients with aphasia may not be able to demonstrate their true decision-making abilities as a result of their language impairments (Suleman and Hopper, 2016).

According to the (Department of Health, 2005), for a person to have capacity about a specific decision at a particular point in time, they must demonstrate ability to:

1. understand the information relevant to the decision,
2. retain that information,
3. use or weigh up that information as part of the process of making the decision, and
4. communicate their decision (whether by talking, using sign language, or any other means).

The Department of Health (2005) states that provision should be in place to ensure that a patient is able to understand the information relevant to the decision. This includes ensuring that information is presented in the most accessible way, optimising a patient's ability to engage fully in the decision-making process. Without this support, patients with communication difficulties are left vulnerable and at risk of decisions being made on their behalf. Two key principles of the Mental Capacity Act are that patients are assumed to have capacity unless it is established otherwise, and that 'a person is not to be treated as unable to make a decision unless all practicable steps to help him to do so have been taken without success'.

Studies have found that people with aphasia are often presumed to lack capacity, leading to potentially unsafe discharges and decisions about health care that do not reflect the patient's choice (Carling-Rowland and Wahl, 2010; Mackenzie et al., 2008). The presence of aphasia has been shown to heighten the presumption of incapacity, highlighting the importance of a skilled and comprehensive assessment process.

Optimising participation in mental capacity assessments for patients with communication difficulties can be challenging, but not impossible. It is important to consider the patient's specific speech or language impairment, and there is no 'one size fits all' approach. The Mental Capacity Code of Practice suggests that capacity assessments should be carried out by the most appropriate person for the decision being made, and that SLTs' skills should be utilised to support those with communication difficulties. Within rehabilitation settings decisions can often be complex, both due to the cognitive and communication challenges faced by patients, and the complexity of the decisions to be made. It is therefore essential to utilise the skills of all members of the IDT when supporting patients to make decisions.

A key factor in maximising a person's ability to engage with the assessment process is time and preparation. SLTs are trained to assess communication impairments in detail, identifying patients' verbal and nonverbal skills, and developing methods of supporting communication using a range of modalities. They also have specific skills in adapting style and means of communication to maximise patients' abilities to engage in the assessment process. However, all members of the IDT have a role to play. The following example illustrates how interdisciplinary working, supported by speech and language therapy guidance, can be used to facilitate effective assessment of mental capacity.

## Case study 4: Supporting a mental capacity assessment

Mrs. G was admitted to a rehabilitation setting following a large subarachnoid haemorrhage. She presented with severe expressive and receptive aphasia and apraxia of speech. It was difficult for occupational therapists and psychologists to fully explore her cognitive skills due to the extent of her communication impairments, however, she presented with reduced attention and some right-sided neglect within functional tasks.

Mrs. G's expressive speech was limited to one or two words which she used repetitively without any meaning, however, she used facial expression and intonation to communicate her message. For example, it was clear whether she intended her output to be a question or a statement. She was able to repeat words inconsistently but initiation did not improve throughout her admission. On assessment, she presented with significant difficulties with understanding spoken and written information, however would often use the context and nonverbal cues to follow a basic conversation.

A number of different communication modalities were used to try to support Mrs. G. With practice she was able to recognise single words when read aloud, and her ability to link pictures to their meaning improved with therapy. She also responded well to photographs and everyday objects. A picture-based communication app was introduced using Mrs. G's iPad and her ability to use this to express daily needs improved with practice. Mrs. G's 'yes' and 'no' response was variable. She would often nod her head whilst putting her thumb down, or shake her head whilst pointing to a 'YES' card. Using too many modalities was confusing for Mrs. G and it was therefore important to strip this back.

Mrs. G also had a high level of physical care needs and it was anticipated that she would need to be discharged to a 24-hour care setting. However, as discharge approached, she began to indicate that she wanted to go home. She had an extremely supportive family but lived alone, therefore being discharged home would mean being left alone for long periods of the day between care calls. She was unable to get to the toilet without carers and therefore would need to use a pad and risk incontinence.

The team and Mrs. G's family had significant concerns about this however acknowledged her wishes and began the complex process of assessing her capacity to make this decision. As the decision was relating to discharge destination, it would ultimately be down to Mrs. G's social worker to determine whether she was able to make this decision, however the input of the IDT was essential. In the weeks prior to the assessments, physiotherapists and occupational therapists spent time explaining to Mrs. G what the options and implications would be regarding transfers and equipment at home. They completed an environmental visit and then a home visit to allow Mrs. G to experience the reality of her home environment. Speech and language therapy support was provided to facilitate this information being presented in the most accessible format. Photographs, key words, and gestures were used to maximise Mrs. G's understanding. This information was given on more than one occasion to help her to retain the key points.

Clinical psychology explored Mrs. G's understanding of the potential impact of independent living on her mood and emotional wellbeing. Joint sessions were completed with SLTs to support communication, using visual scales and emotions pictures on Mrs. G's iPad.

Nursing staff worked with Mrs. G to explore options regarding incontinence. They provided advice about restricting fluid intake in the evenings and, with Mrs. G's consent, replicated the care calls that she would receive at home in order to help her understand what this would feel like.

Mrs. G's family was also involved throughout. The rehabilitation coordinator was key in ensuring that their views and opinions were heard and taken into account. They also liaised closely with the social worker to ensure that all information and any new concerns were communicated between the team.

This 'preassessment' phase took place over a number of weeks and was equally as important as the assessment itself. The information provided in this time contributed significantly to Mrs. G's understanding of the 'full picture' of what the various discharge options would look like.

The social worker and SLT then met a number of times in preparation for the actual assessment. They discussed the questions that the social worker needed to ask Mrs. G, and the key information that she needed her to be able to express. The SLT then prepared materials to support the assessment process. Several sessions were required to complete a comprehensive assessment and Mrs. G's son was present throughout. Assessments were completed in a quiet environment to maximise her attention, and other therapy sessions that day were reduced to limit the impact of fatigue.

Talking Mats (https://www.talkingmats.com) were used to determine Mrs. G's understanding of her abilities and limitations (Talking Mats, n.d.). She sorted a range of simple pictures into two categories, 'HELP' and 'NO HELP' (Fig. 10.3) demonstrating her awareness of current impairments and the areas that she may need assistance with at home. This was used to help guide the rest of the assessment process.

In order to optimise Mrs. G's ability to demonstrate her understanding and communicate a choice, key words were used as options for Mrs. G to tick. It was

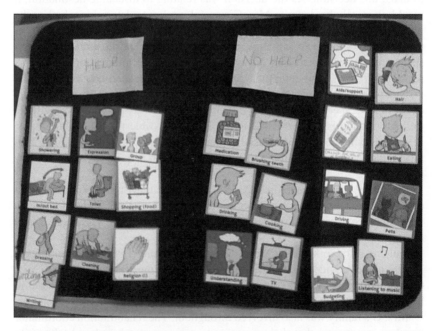

If you were at home, you would have **4 care calls** per day. When you're on your own, would you be able to...

| | |
|---|---|
| Watch the TV | ✓ |
| Get to the toilet | ✗ |
| Talk on the phone | ✗ |
| Listen to music | ✓ |
| Make a hot drink in the kitchen | ✓ |
| Cook a meal | ✗ |
| Answer the front door | ✗ |
| Go out to the shops | ✗ |

**FIGURE 10.4** Examples of written options in a mental capacity assessment.

**RISKS** – at home on your own, do you think you might be at risk of...

| | |
|---|---|
| Feeling lonely | ✗ |
| Forgetting to take medication | ✗ |
| Becoming dehydrated | ✓ |
| Getting hungry | ✗ |
| Feeling bored | ✗ |
| Struggling to call for help in an emergency | ✓ |
| Skin breakdown | ✗ |

**FIGURE 10.5** Examples of written options in a mental capacity assessment.

important to keep language simple whilst establishing the level of detail required for the assessors to make a decision about capacity. Written options were also read aloud, with Mrs. G ticking the ones that she agreed with. Some examples are shown in Figs. 10.4 and 10.5.

A further session was required to increase the level of detail, exploring Mrs. G's understanding of the potential consequences of some of the 'compromises' that she may have to make in order to return home; particularly access to the toilet. Again, using adapted communication strategies (pictures, photographs, key words, and gestures) Mrs. G was able to demonstrate that she understood these issues and communicate her choice to go home. The social worker deemed that Mrs. G had been able to demonstrate the capacity to understand the information regarding the decision, use this information to weigh up the options, and clearly communicate her decision.

The assessment process was a long one and involved many members of the IDT, however, it was important that the process was not rushed, and that Mrs. G's significant communication difficulties did not lead to a presumption of incapacity. With the right support and adaptations, she was able to participate fully in the decision-making process and make an informed choice regarding her discharge destination.

## Assistive technology and alternative and augmentative communication

Assistive technology (AT) refers to any form of equipment that makes life easier and helps people to be more independent. It is any form of software, hardware, or system that helps a person to maintain, improve, or increase their capabilities (Ace Centre, https://acecentre.org.uk/).

In today's society it is common for households to utilise a number of assistive technologies, from hi-tech ways to turn the heating on from your phone and doorbells that allow us to see who is there, even when we're away on holiday, to more simple gadgets that help us to grip and open a jar. These items are becoming increasingly commonplace, and for patients with physical, cognitive, or communication difficulties, they increase opportunities for independence.

It is beyond the scope of this chapter to discuss the many different assistive technologies available, and new ideas are constantly being introduced, however, the following principles apply when considering the use of AT for patients with cognitive and/or communication needs.

1. It is important to make sure the technology is supporting the person and not restricting them. It is also a good idea to look at the person's living space and see if there are adaptations to the environment that may help (e.g., lighting).
2. Consider the degree and types of difficulties the person has—a specific technology might be capable of complex actions, but does the person have the cognitive ability to use it?
3. What are the person's needs, preferences, and ability to use devices? Consider how these may change over time?
4. Does the person have any other conditions that may affect how they use the technology (such as poor sight or hearing)?
5. Do they have support from family, friends, or carers?
6. Will the technology fit in with the person's daily routines, or act as a restriction?

7. Does the technology require a phone line or internet access, and what are the cost implications of this? (Adapted from https://www.alzhiemers.org.uk.)

Alternative and augmentative communication (AAC) is a form of AT to support people with communication difficulties. It has been defined by the International Society for Alternative and Augmentative Communication as:

> 'AAC is a set of tools and strategies that an individual uses to solve everyday communicative challenges. Communication can take many forms such as: speech, a shared glance, text, gestures, facial expressions, touch, sign language, symbols, pictures, speech-generating devices, etc. Everyone uses multiple forms of communication, based upon the context and our communication partner. Effective communication occurs when the intent and meaning of one individual is understood by another person. The form is less important than the successful understanding of the message'.

AAC can take many forms, from simple gestures, pictures and pointing, to more complex techniques involving complex computer technology. Some forms of AAC are part of our everyday communication, such as waving 'hello' or using 'thumbs up' to indicate that we are happy with something. Consider being on holiday in a foreign country and pointing to a map or picture to ask a question or make a request. This may be a useful, temporary solution, however some patients rely solely on AAC to facilitate their understanding and/or help them to express themselves.

There is no 'one size fits all' AAC solution when patients present with communication difficulties. It is essential to consider the type and severity of their difficulty and implement a form of AAC that is appropriate for that individual patient. A number of other factors must be considered:

1. Positioning and access
2. Vision
3. Hearing
4. Symbol recognition
5. Verbal language comprehension
6. Reading and spelling abilities
7. Expressive language skills
8. Motivation
9. Fatigue
10. Attention

## Case study 5: Utilising AAC with a communication disorder

The following case study illustrates the AAC journey of a patient with no functional verbal communication following a brain injury:

Miss N was admitted following a severe traumatic brain injury. She had significant physical impairments to both her upper and lower limbs and was dependent on nursing staff to support with all activities of daily living. She was initially nil by mouth with all nutrition, hydration, and medication administered via percutaneous endoscopic gastrostomy. Miss N was able to vocalise in response to pain or discomfort however was unable to produce any purposeful verbal communication. She had a left-sided neglect and found it difficult to maintain her head in a midline position.

Miss N was reluctant to participate in any form of therapeutic activity and would actively disengage from therapists, making it difficult to determine whether there had been any cognitive changes. It had been suggested that Miss N may benefit from use of eye-gaze technology to support her communication and her family were keen to explore this option.

SLTs attempted to complete the preliminary work required to determine whether this was an appropriate option, and what form of software would be most appropriate. Prior to introducing any form of alternative or augmentative communication (AAC), it is essential to determine the patient's level of physical, cognitive, and linguistic abilities.

In this case it was necessary to assess Miss N's level of understanding of symbols and picture material, her ability to read written words, her level of understanding, expressive language and word retrieval, and her ability to spell. Miss N was reluctant to engage with any form of language assessment at this stage; however, her family was keen to go ahead with the eye-gaze trial.

Miss N found it difficult to maintain her head in an upright and midline position. Even with facilitation and support she fatigued quickly, making the calibration process extremely time-consuming and frustrating for Miss N. When she did achieve accurate calibration, the level of control required to accurately position the cursor with eye movements was extremely fatiguing and Miss N would quickly disengage.

This is an example of how hi-tech equipment is not always the most appropriate. Miss N's family had read about this technology and was extremely keen to try it, however without the fundamental skills required to access it, the eye-gaze system was ineffective and frustrating for the patient.

Over time Miss N regained more control in her upper limb and was able to use her right hand to point. With increased trust in staff and improved participation in tasks, it was possible to assess her language skills with more consistency. Miss N demonstrated a good understanding of picture material and was able to use a picture-based communication book to express her basic needs and emotions. Miss N found the hospital environment increasingly difficult to tolerate and it was agreed that discharge home with community therapy and a package of care would be in her best interests at that time.

She continued to be reviewed within the community and continued to make progress, particularly with her cognitive and communication skills. Comprehensive assessment showed that Miss N presented with no specific language impairments, however severe dysarthria and apraxia of speech made speech extremely difficult. She was able to follow complex verbal information and understand written material without difficulty. An alphabet board was introduced to facilitate communication and Miss N was able to use this effectively to spell words. However, this became time-consuming and did not allow Miss N to express herself to the maximum of her language abilities. She was referred to the local specialist centre for communication aids who visited to complete an assessment.

Miss N's head control, visual skills, and fine motor control had improved to a level which allowed her to access a text-based communication app on a large-screen tablet computer. The predictive text function sped up the process and allowed her to use longer and more complex sentence structures. The system was also linked to her social media accounts, allowing her to communicate more effectively with her friends and family. Despite her inability to use speech, Miss N is now able to communicate effectively. She receives regular reviews and equipment is updated as technology improves.

Miss N is also an excellent example of the importance of intervention at the right time and in the right environment. For Miss N, progress was slow and took place over a number of years postinjury. The rehabilitation network model allowed this progress to be monitored closely, and intervention to be provided when most appropriate.

## Summary

This chapter has discussed communication disorders and the impact on a person's wellbeing and rehabilitation journey. We hope that the information, along with the case studies, facilitates learning, and highlights the role of interdisciplinary working in the rehabilitation of patients with communication disorders.

### Reflective questions

- Thinking about a patient, is there something you could change about your practice that would support the patient's communication? How may you implement this?
- What challenges have you faced when completing capacity assessments with patients with communication difficulties? Would you do anything differently now?
- What advice might you give to families?
- What factors would you need to consider when thinking about AAC for somebody with communication difficulties?

## References

Aphasia. National Institute on Deafness and Other Communication Disorders (NIDCD), 2010. Available at: https://www.nidcd.nih.gov/health/aphasia. Accessed October 7, 2021.

Appelbaum, P.S., Grisso, T., 1988. Assessing patients' capacities to consent to treatment. New Engl. J. Med. 319 (25), 1635–1638.

Bloodstein, O., Bernstein Ratner, N., 2008. A Handbook on Stuttering. Thomson Delmar Learning, Clifton Park, NY.

Brown, K., Worrall, L.E., Davidson, B., Howe, T., 2012. Living successfully with aphasia: a qualitative meta-analysis of the perspectives of individuals with aphasia, family members, and speech-language pathologists. Int. J. Speech Lang. Pathol. 14 (2), 141–155.

Carling-Rowland, A., Wahl, J., 2010. The evaluation of capacity to make admission decisions: is it a fair process for individuals with communication barriers? Med. Law Int. 10 (3), 171–190.

Code, C., 2003. Aphasia Recovery, Treatment and Psychological Adjustment. Cambridge University Press. Available at: https://www.cambridge.org/core. Accessed February 1, 2020. Cambridge Books Online 2009.

Gleason, J.B., 2001. The Development of Language. Pearson Education, Boston.

Jumonville, A., Collins, J.W., O'Brien, N.P., 2012. The Greenwood Dictionary of Education, second ed. Greenwood Press, Santa Barbara, CA 2011.

Kay, J., Lesser, R., Coltheart, M., 1996. Psycholinguistic assessments of language processing in aphasia (PALPA): an introduction. Aphasiology 10 (2), 159–180. doi:10.1080/02687039608248403. www.tandfonline.com.

Mackenzie, J., Lincoln, N., Newby, G., 2008. Capacity to make a decision about discharge destination after stroke: a pilot study. Clin. Rehab. 22 (12), 1116–1126.

Maher, L.M., Clayton, M.C., Barrett, A.M., Schober-Peterson, D., Rothi, L.G.J., 1998. Rehabilitation of a case of pure alexia: exploiting residual abilities. J. Int. Neuropsychol. Soc. 4 (6), 636–647.

Mental Capacity Act. Department of Health, 2005. Available at: https://www.gov.uk/government/organisations/department-of-health-and-social-care. Accessed February 1, 2020.

Nordquist, R., 2019. Orality: definition and examples. ThoughtCo. Available at: https://www.thoughtco.com/orality-communication-term-1691455. Accessed February 1, 2020.

Simmons-Mackie, N., Savage, M., Worrall, L., 2014. Conversation therapy for aphasia: a qualitative review of the literature. Int. J. Lang. Commun. Disord. 49 (5), 511–526.

Suleman, S., Hopper, T., 2016. Decision-making capacity and aphasia: speech-language pathologists' perspectives. Aphasiology 30 (4), 381–395.

Talking Mats. (n.d.). Talking Mats | Improving communication, improving lives. [online] Available at: https://www.talkingmats.com. Accessed February 1, 2020.

# Chapter 11

# Dysphagia in rehabilitation: an interdisciplinary approach

Elaine Bailey and Lisa Barklin

## Chapter outline

## Abstract

Approximately 8% of the world's population is affected by a swallowing disorder, known as dysphagia (Chichero et al., cited by Lecko, 2014). The swallow is a complex set of mechanisms, and a difficulty can occur at any stage of the process. An unsafe swallow can result in a patient becoming medically unwell, which can at times, be fatal. Dysphagia will occur in many disease situations, and patients admitted to specialist rehabilitation settings can present with symptoms that vary significantly in aetiology, prognosis, severity, and presentation. If dysphagia is not managed effectively, rehabilitation may be prolonged, impacting on a patient's ability to reach their maximum rehabilitation potential. Managing dysphagia and making decisions regarding nutrition and hydration can be complex and challenging. Speech and language therapists work closely with other members of the interdisciplinary team to identify and implement strategies and techniques to maximise safety for patients with dysphagia. Ethical dilemmas are frequent,

A Practical Approach to Interdisciplinary Complex Rehabilitation.
DOI: https://doi.org/10.1016/B978-0-7020-8276-4.00011-4

and shared decision making and patient engagement are fundamental in dysphagia management. An interdisciplinary approach is central in contributing to positive outcomes, and allowing positive risk taking and increased opportunity in a safe, interdisciplinary environment.

**Keywords**
Dysphagia; Rehabilitation; Interdisciplinary management; Ethical decision making; Best interest; Mental capacity

## Aims and objectives

The aim of this chapter is to discuss the impact of dysphagia on the rehabilitation journey and the positive influence that interdisciplinary team (IDT) working has on a patient's outcome.

## Overview

The chapter will first provide a basic understanding of what dysphagia is, how common it is, and what causes it. We will consider the physiology and cortical control of swallowing and the impact that this may have on rehabilitation. We will consider why dysphagia is an issue, understanding the risks and consequences. We will look at how interdisciplinary working influences positive outcomes. The chapter will also consider the areas of ethics and mental capacity in patients presenting with dysphagia, as well as positive risk taking and increased opportunity in a safe, interdisciplinary environment.

## Definition

Firstly, we need to understand what we mean by dysphagia. The word 'dysphagia' is derived from Greek, with 'dys' meaning disorders and 'phagein' meaning to eat (Groher and Crary, 2010). Logemann (1998) describes dysphagia as 'an absence or impairment of the swallowing process due to weakness, incoordination, damage, or surgery to the muscles or structures used for swallowing'. Swallowing and breathing are intimately related as they both share the same path, but as they pass through the pharynx, air enters the larynx, and food and liquid continues to the oesophagus. When this relationship is disturbed, swallowing problems and dysphagia occur (Matsuo et al., 2008).

## Incidence

Approximately 8% of the world's population is affected by dysphagia. In the developed world this amounts to 99 million individuals (Chichero et al., cited by Lecko, 2014). The presentation of dysphagia will depend on the context in which it occurs. The commonest complaints will be that food and liquid goes down the wrong way into the lungs rather than into the stomach. In individuals who cannot recognise or communicate their problem, coughing, food refusal, regurgitation, and spitting may be the presenting concern observed by carers (Smithard, 2015).

An unsafe swallow can result in a patient becoming medically unwell, which can, at times, be fatal. Dysphagic symptoms may result in aspiration (the entry of material below the level of the vocal cords), aspiration pneumonia, choking, dehydration and malnutrition, oral infections, reduced stamina and physical ability, chronic pain, increased hospital admission, and reduced psychological wellbeing.

'Effective swallowing is essential for parts of human life, satiety, and pleasure, and is one of the most important aspects of social life' (Kjaersgaard, 2013). Food is part of our identity that we carry with us (Bourdieu, 1992). Dysphagia is an important issue related to a patient's quality of life and the ability to eat safely together with others (Johansson and Johansson, 2009).

## Mechanism of swallowing

*Cortical control of swallowing*

Swallowing is a complex neuromuscular sequence of events that depends on a hierarchical interaction between the cerebral cortex, the brain stem, and cranial nerves (Mistry and Hamdy, 2008). The main centre for swallowing control is located in the brain stem and has two functions: to trigger and time the swallow pattern, and to control the motor neurons involved in swallowing (Gonzalez-Fernandez and Daniels, 2008). It is difficult to tease out the precise areas involved in cortical control of swallowing. Patients can have the same aetiology but present with different symptoms. Evidence shows that swallowing musculature is bilaterally controlled and independent of handedness (Ertekin and Aydogdu, 2003). This may explain why some patients present with dysphagia following a neurological event, and why some will retain or regain a safe swallow (Singh and Hamdy, 2006). Ertekin (2011) states that a voluntary swallow and a reflexive swallow differ in the origin of the swallow trigger. This means that whilst a patient may be able to perform a swallow to command, they may still struggle to reflexively swallow food and/or fluid safely. Volitional swallowing occurs with the desire to eat, reflexive swallowing occurs as a result of saliva or food remnants in the mouth. Volitional swallowing is part of eating behaviour and is planned, reflexive swallowing is a protective reflexive action (Ertekin, 2011).

Healthy people swallow approximately once every minute. This frequency decreases with normal ageing (Logemann, 1998). Swallowing is a complex function in which food and liquid are transported from the oral cavity to the stomach as a well-coordinated function (Miller, 2008). It is estimated that 26 pairs of muscles are used in the swallow process, along with five cranial nerves (Mistry and Hamdy, 2008). To better understand dysphagia, we first need to understand the normal physiology of eating and swallowing (Matsuo and Palmer, 2008).

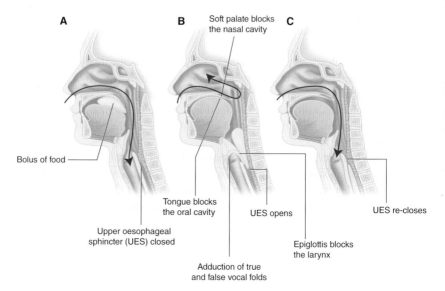

FIGURE 11.1 (A–C) Stages of swallowing. From Sun, N., Tsang R., 2019. Oropharinx anatomy and physiology of swallowing. In: Kuipers E (Ed). *Encyclopedia of Gastroenterology*. 2nd ed. AP/Elsevier, 748–756.

Swallowing consists of four stages:

1. Preoral stage (voluntary)
2. Oral stage (voluntary)
3. Pharyngeal stage (involuntary)
4. Oesophageal stage (involuntary)

We will discuss these stages in a small amount of detail. It is not the purpose of this chapter to teach the anatomy and physiology of the swallow, only to provide an overview. Further reading will be required should the reader wish to expand their knowledge of the normal swallow (Fig. 11.1).

Below is a basic description of the phases:

1. *Preoral stage*: A state of readiness for eating—feeling hungry or thirsty, discussing food, choosing food, smelling food, anticipation, posture. 'Setting the scene' for the next stage (Coombes, 2011). This stage is voluntary.
2. *Oral stage*: Takes 1–20 seconds and involves mastication in order to form the food into a bolus. This stage is also voluntary and the airway remains open in order to breathe in and out of the nose.
3. *Pharyngeal stage*: This stage is a reflex and is therefore involuntary. Breathing stops during this stage. The bolus moves over the back of the tongue, enters the pharynx, and moves down towards the top of the oesophageal sphincter.
4. *Oesophageal stage*: This stage is also involuntary and involves the bolus entering the oesophagus and being transported to the stomach.

**TABLE 11.1** Aetiology and examples.

| Aetiology | Examples |
| --- | --- |
| Neurological | Hypoxic and traumatic head injury, brain tumour, stroke, Parkinson's disease, multiple sclerosis, motor neuron disease, Huntington's disease, dementia, Guillain Barre syndrome, myasthenia gravis |
| Structural | Tumour of the head and neck, oral cancer, benign strictures such as pouches or webs, ulcers, lack of dentition, infection |
| Respiratory | Tracheostomy (although it should be noted that not all patients with a tracheostomy will present with dysphagia), pneumonia, COPD, and any diseases that raise the respiratory rate. Swallowing requires a period of apnoea, and where this is not possible, dysphagia may occur |
| Cognitive | Reduced perceptual and cognitive awareness of the eating situation, hence reduced physiological responses (Leopold and Kagel, 1996), e.g., recognition of food |
| Psychological | Globus, fear, anxiety, avoidance |
| Complicating factors | Communication difficulties, alertness levels, poor posture, poor oral hygiene. |
| Ageing | In those people who are frail, the swallowing only becomes a problem when another stressor such as infection or medication wipes out their physiological reserve resulting in dysphagia and the risk of aspiration (Smithard, 2015) |

## Causes of dysphagia

Dysphagia will occur in many disease situations (see Table 11.1 for examples), not just in the presence of neurological disease. Patients admitted to specialist rehabilitation settings can present with symptoms of dysphagia which vary significantly in aetiology, prognosis, severity, and presentation. Dysphagia can occur in isolation, however, this is very rarely the case. More often than not, swallowing difficulties co-occur with complex physical, cognitive, and/or communication difficulties. The table is not exhaustive but is intended to provide the reader with an understanding of the types of causes of dysphagia.

The approach to the management of dysphagia will be dependent on the cause, and whether the disease process is expected to progress or improve.

## Assessment of dysphagia

Assessment of dysphagia includes both subjective bedside assessment and objective instrumental assessments.

### Bedside assessment

A bedside dysphagia assessment involves a physical examination of the oro-musculature, followed by a detailed assessment of the patient's ability to swallow food and fluid of different consistencies, whilst observing for signs of difficulty. The preoral, oral, pharyngeal, and oesophageal stages of swallowing are assessed. Factors such as oral transit time, initiation of swallowing, laryngeal elevation, spillage, residue, condition of swallow, laryngeal closure, reflux, aspiration, and ability to clear residue are monitored. Where a bedside assessment is inconclusive in determining the risk of aspiration and the safety of the swallow, an objective assessment is then considered.

## Cervical auscultation

Cervical Auscultation (CA) involves the use of a stethoscope, placed on the patient's throat to listen to the sounds of the swallow. Trained clinicians use CA to assess swallow and airway sounds. This allows the clinician to judge whether the swallow presents as within normal limits, or determine the degree of impairment of swallowing. CA is usually used as an adjunct to bedside assessment.

## Videofluoroscopy

Videofluoroscopy is a radiological examination used to study the oral, pharyngeal, and oesophageal stages of swallowing. It identifies aspiration and swallowing problems on an X-ray. It is also used in determining the success of dietary and compensatory strategies. The assessment is carried out by providing food types of different consistencies, whilst factors such as oral transit time, initiation of swallowing, laryngeal elevation, spillage, residue, condition of swallow, laryngeal closure, reflux, aspiration, and ability to clear residue are monitored. (The terms videofluoroscopic swallowing study [videofluoroscopy] and modified barium swallow are often used interchangeably).

## Fibreoptic endoscopic evaluation of swallowing

Fibreoptic endoscopic evaluation of swallowing is an alternative to videofluoroscopic examination of patients at risk of aspiration. The procedure entails passing a flexible endoscope into the oropharynx. Evaluation is carried out by providing food types of different consistencies whilst factors such as oral transit time, initiation of swallowing, laryngeal elevation, spillage, residue, condition of swallow, laryngeal closure, reflux, aspiration, and ability to clear residue are monitored.

## The effect of dysphagia on the rehabilitation journey

If dysphagia is not managed effectively, this may result in unnecessary prolonged rehabilitation and inappropriate transfers between acute and rehabilitation units (Kjaersgaard, 2013). Frequent and prolonged periods with infection will result in reduced medical status and reduced stamina. This will adversely affect a patient's ability to engage in meaningful rehabilitation programmes, prolonging the rehabilitation process (Perry and Love, 2001; Westergren, 2006) and thereby impacting on the patient's ability to reach their maximum rehabilitation potential. Minimising the risks and episodes of aspiration, maximising nutritional intake, and providing the patient with the most appropriate oral feeding will help to facilitate the maximal recovery potential for individuals (Mackay et al., 1999).

## Rationale for IDT working

Whilst speech and language therapists are recognised as being the experts in assessment, diagnosis, and management of dysphagia, it is the interdisciplinary approach that further contributes to positive outcomes. Frontline clinicians are in a unique position to be alert to the high prevalence of swallowing difficulty among patients, to evaluate and identify those who need assessment, and assure that individuals are appropriately treated (Cichero et al., 2009). IDTs are more effectively able to manage dysphagia, reduce the economic and social burden, and improve patients' quality of life. Rehabilitation settings with an interdisciplinary approach attain significantly better patient outcomes including reduced cases of pneumonia (by 55%) and reduced hospital length of stay (Cichero et al., 2009). Successful mealtime experiences require functioning of multiple areas that go beyond the swallow itself, such as adequate visual field, optimal positioning, fine-motor skills for self-feeding, functional sitting balance with sustained abilities to complete meals, cognitive and language skills to attend to the task of oral intake and follow directions, and oral, pharyngeal, and oesophageal function for safe and adequate intake (Kinder, 2016).

## Interdisciplinary management of dysphagia

Managing dysphagia and making decisions regarding nutrition and hydration can be complex and challenging, both for the patient and their family and for the treating team of clinicians. As speech and language therapists working in specialist rehabilitation, the primary goal of intervention for patients with dysphagia is to maximise their ability to eat and drink orally. Oral intake, modified as necessary, should be the main aim of treatment (RCP Guidelines, 2010). 'Patients with oral feeding difficulties deserve special care but may not always receive it. Their care should be tailored to their requirements, not to the needs of others, and should, as far as possible, preserve their oral intake' (RCP Guidelines, 2010).

There are a range of strategies used to support patients with dysphagia, many of which do not require any direct modification of their diet or fluids. Speech and language therapists work closely with other members of the IDT to identify and implement strategies and techniques to optimise the mealtime experience, and maximise safety for patients with dysphagia.

### Environment

Mealtimes are extremely important in preserving cultural and social identity (Atkinson and O'Kane, 2018). Changes to mealtime patterns such as an unfamiliar environment, dependence on others and modified diet or fluids can all impact on a patient's oral intake (Aselage and Amella, 2010). An individual approach to managing mealtimes within the rehabilitation setting is vital, and the benefits of adjusting and optimising the mealtime environment should not be underestimated. This is particularly the case for patients with cognitive and/or communication difficulties. Patients with cognitive or sensory deficits may be disorientated to time or place, limiting their ability to access information that facilitates the preoral stage of the swallow. Providing prompts about time of day, introducing appealing smells, or engaging in practical tasks such as setting the table can help to support some of these difficulties.

For some patients with cognitive difficulties, eating in a busy dining room setting can be overwhelming and overstimulating, reducing their ability to attend to their meal, and potentially impacting on the safety of their oral intake. For these patients, reducing background noise, removing distractions (e.g., turning off the television), and limiting interruptions at mealtimes are important (Cleary et al., 2009), and nursing staff play a key role in identifying and facilitating environmental changes. For patients with communication difficulties, social settings at mealtimes can be daunting and are often described as a source of anxiety. The prospect of being unable to fully engage in a mealtime conversation may result in a patient selecting to eat in isolation. Rehabilitation nursing staff play a key role in ensuring that individual patient need is recognised, and that all patients are given a choice about their mealtime preferences. Within an inpatient rehabilitation setting, nursing staff are available to provide a 24-hour approach, and are ideally placed to identify patients with swallowing problems, and implement interdisciplinary guidelines to ensure that the patient receives the best possible opportunity for safe nutrition and hydration.

Conversely, a more social setting can be extremely helpful in engaging patients in the mealtime experience. For some patients, particularly those with cognitive impairments, eating in isolation at their bedside is unfamiliar and 'unnatural'. They may find it difficult to initiate eating independently or refuse to eat at all. This increases their level of dependence and need for support from staff. Many of these patients benefit from the social interaction of eating with other people in a 'dining room' setting, as they are automatically surrounded by sensory feedback and social cues, which in turn can prompt initiation of the familiar actions of eating and drinking. This can lead to increased independence and improved oral intake without the need for direct intervention from staff.

## Physical and sensory impairments

Physiotherapists and occupational therapists play an important role in optimising posture and positioning for patients with dysphagia. Postural control is recognised as being fundamental to selective normal movement patterns for all activities, including movements of the face and oral tract, therefore postural control is an integral part of dysphagia treatment (Coombes, 2011). Ideally patients should be sat in an upright, midline position to maximise the safety of their swallow, however, many patients are unable to achieve this independently following a traumatic illness or injury. They may require supportive seating to maintain their posture once out of bed, or specific handling in order to achieve a safe, upright position.

Patients with spinal braces require an interdisciplinary approach to their dysphagia management. It is essential to follow specific spinal guidelines regarding restrictions to range of movement, in order to avoid further harm. Such guidelines often involve limiting the angle at which patients are allowed to sit upright, making it challenging to achieve an optimal positioning for eating and drinking. Cervical collars can also extend the neck into an unnatural, and potentially unsafe, position for eating and drinking. Some designs may also interfere with the laryngeal prominence (or 'Adam's apple'), restricting hyolaryngeal movement or causing pain/discomfort on swallowing. It is essential that speech and language therapists work alongside orthotists, physiotherapists, occupational therapists, and nurses to ensure that swallowing safety is optimised within the limitations of spinal guidelines.

Following significant illness or injury, many rehabilitation patients present with physical or sensory deficits which limit their ability to feed themselves independently. Patients with upper limb weakness may require assistance with cutting food or bringing food to their mouth. This loss of control can lead to patients feeling vulnerable or frustrated. Rehabilitation nurses are skilled in supporting and encouraging patients to be as independent as possible. They are also sensitive to those feelings of vulnerability and frustration, providing empathetic support when direct intervention is required. Patients with dysphagia who are dependent for feeding are at greater risk of developing aspiration pneumonia than those who are independent (McGrail et al., 2012). Strategies such as 'hand over hand feeding' can be beneficial in supporting patients with more complex physical needs. This involves the patient holding the cutlery, with the person providing support placing their hand over the patient's hand and guiding its movement. Facilitating arm and hand movement provides additional information to the brain about the task and may prompt subsequent stages of the swallow (Shune et al., 2016). Occupational therapists can provide advice about specific equipment that may increase independence with eating and drinking, such as adapted cutlery and plateguards.

Rehabilitation patients often present with sensory deficits such as visual loss or inattention. They require additional support to maximise their oral intake, such as ensuring that cutlery or drinks are placed on their unaffected side, prompting them to attend to both sides of their plate.

## Communication

Patients with communication difficulties also require particular consideration. They may lack initiation or find it difficult to communicate when they are hungry or thirsty, increasing their risk of malnutrition or dehydration (consequences of this are discussed further in Chapter 12—Nutrition and dietetics in rehabilitation). Consider a patient who consistently nods when offered, but then refuses to drink every cup of tea that is brought to them throughout the day, resulting in significant concern about their fluid intake. With support using a picture-based communication book, you discover that the patient dislikes tea and will only drink coffee, but is unable to express this verbally. Ensuring that patients have an effective method of communicating food and drink choices is extremely important, and the role of catering staff cannot be underestimated. Speech and language therapists work closely with the catering team in order to ensure that patients can clearly communicate their choices, using picture menus or closed questions where necessary. Training has also been effective in raising catering staff's awareness of the potential consequences of dysphagia and increasing their confidence when implementing speech and language therapy recommendations.

### Diet and fluid modifications

Strategies such as those described above may often be sufficient to support patients with dysphagia, but in many cases a more direct modification of diet and/or fluid recommendations is required. The success of these recommendations requires considerable patient participation and compliance (Kaizer et al., 2012). Many patients, capable of feeding themselves independently, are compliant with specific speech and language therapy recommendations, however, Sharp and Bryant (2003) suggest that as many as 40% are not. Correlation has been suggested between the level of compliance and the type of modification suggested, with patients more likely to adhere to recommendations for modification to diet than fluids (Low et al., 2001). See Fig. 11.2 for descriptions of diet and fluid modifications.

Diet and fluid modification are widely used strategies within speech and language therapy practice, however, there is a growing body of evidence which questions its effectiveness. Clinical experience suggests that in many cases, diet and/or fluid modification is successful in preventing patients from harm, however at what cost to their quality of life? There is a lack of quality evidence in the literature to support the benefit of modified diet and fluids (O'Keefe, 2018) highlighting the need for further research to inform clinical practice. In the absence of such research, it is important for clinicians to use the evidence that is available to them, whilst taking a person-centred approach to dysphagia management in individual patients.

### Medical management

Medical teams consider how medication may interact with dysphagia symptoms; for example, some medications may be too thin and pose an aspiration risk, some may cause xerostomia (dry mouth) or have sedating properties. Medical teams

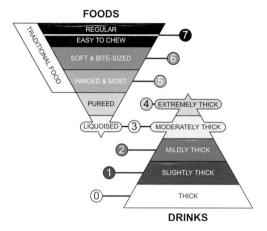

FIGURE 11.2    International dysphagia diet standardisation initiative. © The International Dysphagia Diet Standardisation Initiative 2019 @ https://iddsi.org/framework.

and physiotherapists are able to monitor and manage a patient's chest in order to identify any change in chest status.

## Pharmacy

If a patient is taking tablets with thickened fluids, a pharmacist should always be consulted, as gum-based thickeners have been shown to affect the release and absorption of some medications (Cichero, 2013). A pharmacist and prescriber must be consulted before manipulating the form of any medication (Atkinson and O'Kane, 2018).

With the support of the IDT, as discussed above, speech and language therapists are more able to increase therapeutic opportunities for patients admitted to the rehabilitation unit. An example of this is demonstrated in case study 1 below.

---

**Case study 1**

Mr. N was admitted following a traumatic brain injury. He was nil by mouth on admission with all nutrition, hydration, and medication administered via his enteral feeding tube. Mr. N was desperate to eat and drink, and being nil by mouth had a significant impact on his mood and motivation. Being in active rehabilitation with the availability of the IDT allowed speech and language therapists to take positive risks within a supported environment. Physiotherapists and occupational therapists worked to optimise seating and positioning. The team worked together to minimise fatigue during the day and developed a routine for sitting out that incorporated mealtimes. As oral trials commenced, physiotherapists

*(continued)*

> **Case study 1 — cont'd**
>
> and medical staff closely monitored Mr. N's chest status. As Mr. N was increasingly able to manage his secretions, medical staff discontinued his anticholinergic medications, with a notable improvement in his level of alertness. Mr. N's oral intake was gradually increased; speech and language therapists worked alongside dietetic colleagues to adjust his enteral feeding regimen, optimising his appetite whilst ensuring that his nutritional needs were met. Nursing staff were closely involved in optimising Mr. N's environment and providing prompting during mealtimes as required. Mr. N made excellent progress during his rehabilitation; he was discharged on normal diet and fluids and no longer required his feeding tube.

## Managing risk

A frequent challenge for clinicians working in rehabilitation settings are those patients with dysphagia who choose not to accept advice regarding diet and fluid recommendations. Patients in active rehabilitation often face significant challenges—loss of role, increased dependency, change in social or family status—and additionally restricting their choices about eating and drinking can impact negatively on their quality of life (McCurtin et al., 2018).

Ethical decision making in dysphagia may often be associated with patients receiving end-of-life care. It is uncommon to face such decisions within active rehabilitation, however, ethical dilemmas remain frequent. It is important to consider what we are trying to achieve; to sustain life, improve quality of life, or prioritise safety? Is it possible to achieve all of these simultaneously?

Shared decision making and patient engagement are fundamental in dysphagia management. As speech and language therapists, our role is to assess and make recommendations, but also to educate the patient and their family about the potential risks and rationale for any advice provided. Without this, patients and/or families may feel they are forced to follow a dysphagia management plan that they do not understand or agree with, increasing the risk that patients will not follow recommendations. It is essential to listen to individual patients and their own views regarding 'risk'. As clinicians it is important to acknowledge our own attitudes and beliefs towards 'risk' and prevent these from biasing our own decision making.

When patients choose to take what are assessed to be 'risks', it can be ethically challenging for clinicians. As health care professionals, our aim is to promote wellbeing and minimise the likelihood of harm. Within clinical practice we are taught to prioritise patient safety, with the perception that risk is closely linked to concepts of accountability and blame (Atwal et al., 2011). However, prioritising safety and promoting overall wellbeing are not always black and white concepts and the two may result in conflicting recommendations. Such situations may be sources of moral unease or distress for health care profession-als (Browne, 2003). These concerns may be elevated if they feel they are active participants in an activity that places the patient at risk of serious harm, such as feeding patients or providing their meals.

When patients do not follow speech and language therapy guidelines, it is essential to consider their ability to make an informed decision. Clinical practice is guided by the Mental Capacity Act (2005), which protects patient autonomy and their right and ability to make an informed choice. Speech and language therapists are frequently involved in mental capacity assessments for patients with dysphagia. It is our responsibility to ensure that the patient understands their swallowing difficulty and the potential risks associated with this, and to explain the rationale for any recommendations provided. Assessments can often be challenging and are rarely 'clear-cut'. Patients are often able to describe the risks as they have been presented to them, however struggle to implement these in practice or feel that 'it will not happen to them'.

If patients are deemed to lack the capacity to make decisions regarding their eating and drinking, a 'best interests' decision must be made. It is important to ensure that the patient's family fully understand the information provided and that the views of the patient are taken into consideration. For each alternative option it is important to consider the risks versus the benefits and determine the 'least restrictive' option. It may be that clinicians have significant concerns about a particular outcome, however, these may be outweighed by a patient's expressed wishes.

Such situations can be a 'stressful and emotionally demanding experience for the team; an experience that is commonly reported by health professionals when making best interests decisions on behalf of someone else' (Williams et al., 2014). Where patients lack the capacity to make these decisions and take these risks for themselves, it is down to the treating team, along with the family, to make recommendations in the patient's best interests; but there is often no definitive 'right answer'. We have a level of professional responsibility to ensure our patients' wellbeing that goes beyond simply 'keeping them safe', however making such decisions in practice is challenging. In the Court of Protection case, Local Authority X v MM & Anor (No. 1) (2007), Judge Munby stated, 'the fact is that all life involves risk….physical health and safety can sometimes be bought at too high a price in happiness and emotional welfare….the emphasis must be on sensible risk appraisal…what good is it making someone safer if it merely makes them miserable?'

The purpose of the above discussion was not to provide answers, as each individual case will be different, but to highlight some of the factors that must be considered when supporting decision making for patients with dysphagia. These can be summarised as:

1. Comprehensive assessment
2. Education and information for patients and families

3. Supported mental capacity assessments (for those patients whose capacity to make the decision is questioned)
4. Supported and shared decision making
5. Consideration of, and respect for, the views of the patient
6. Determination of the least restrictive option

## Key learning points

1. What dysphagia is
2. The mechanism of the normal swallow
3. Causes of dysphagia
4. The effect of dysphagia on the rehabilitation journey
5. Interdisciplinary management of dysphagia
6. Decision making for patients with dysphagia

### Reflective questions

Two clinical scenarios are outlined below. What factors would you need to consider, and what might be the challenges for the patient, their family, and staff?

1. A young patient was admitted for active rehabilitation following hypertensive encephalopathy and right frontal lobe hemorrhage secondary to hypertension. He was nil by mouth on admission with all nutrition, hydration and medication administered via PEG. He presented with severe dysarthria characterised by weak, flaccid movements in the lips and tongue, which made it difficult to break down food textures. Videofluoroscopy assessment showed aspiration on normal fluids. He progressed to tolerating Level 2 fluids and Level 4 (pureed) diet (Fig.11.2 for descriptions), however compliance with Level 4 diet was limited and his oral intake was severely reduced. He was also inconsistent with taking bolus feeds, therefore there were significant concerns about weight loss and nutritional status.

   Mental capacity assessment was completed over a number of sessions. He was provided with verbal and written information about his specific swallowing difficulty and the videofluoroscopy was used to illustrate this. The rationale for recommendations made and the potential risks of not following them were also explained.

   He was consistently able to 'recite' the risks as they had been presented to him, however repeatedly stated, 'but it won't happen to me'.
2. Mrs. B was admitted for active rehabilitation following an inflammatory brainstem lesion. She presented with a vocal cord paralysis and severely impaired upper oesophageal sphincter function, resulting in risk of aspiration on all diet and fluid textures trialed. She was initially nil by mouth with all nutrition, hydration and medication administered via her PEG. Mrs. B fully understood her swallowing difficulties and the potential risks associated with eating and drinking.

She had a young family and would regularly cook for them on home leave.
The family stopped going out together as Mrs. B was unable to eat or drink.

# References

Aselage, M.B., Amella, E.J., 2010. An evolutionary analysis of mealtime difficulties in older adults with dementia. J. Clin. Nurs. 19 (1–2), 33–41.

Atkinson, K., O'Kane, L., 2018. Thickener and beyond: an individualised approach to dysphagia management. Br. J. Neurosci. Nurs. 14 (Suppl. 2), S13–S19.

Atwal, A., Wiggett, C., McIntyre, A., 2011. Risks with older adults in acute care settings: occupational therapists' and physiotherapists' perceptions. Br. J. Occup. Ther. 74 (9), 412–418.

Bourdieu, P., 1992. Distinction: a social critique of the judgement of taste. J. Econ. Sociol. 6 (3), 25–48 [online].

Browne, A., 2003. Helping residents live at risk. Cambridge. Q. Healthc. Ethics 12 (1), 83–90.

Cichero, J.A., 2013. Thickening agents used for dysphagia management: effect on bioavailability of water, medication and feelings of satiety. Nutr. J. 12 (1), 1–8.

Cichero, J.A., Heaton, S., Bassett, L., 2009. Triaging dysphagia: nurse screening for dysphagia in an acute hospital. J. Clin. Nurs. 18 (11), 1649–1659.

Cleary, S., 2009. Using environmental interventions to facilitate eating and swallowing in residents with dementia. Can. Nurs. Home 20 (2), 5–12.

Coombes, K., 2011. ARCOS – Association for Rehabilitation of Communication and Oral Skills. Available at: http://www.arcos.org.uk. Accessed October 7, 2021.

Crary, M.A., Groher, M.E., 2010. Dysphagia : clinical management in adults and children. Mosby, S.L.

Ertekin, C., 2011. Voluntary versus spontaneous swallowing in man. Dysphagia 26 (2), 183–192.

Ertekin, C., Aydogdu, I., 2003. Neurophysiology of swallowing. Clin. Neurophysiol. 114 (12), 2226–2244.

González-Fernández, M., Daniels, S.K., 2008. Dysphagia in stroke and neurologic disease. Phys. Med. Rehab. Clin. North Am. 19 (4), 867–888.

Johansson, A.E.M., Johansson, U., 2009. Relatives' experiences of family members' eating difficulties. Scand. J. Occup. Ther. 16 (1), 25–32.

Kaizer, F., Spiridigliozzi, A.-M., Hunt, M.R., 2012. Promoting shared decision-making in rehabilitation: development of a framework for situations when patients with dysphagia refuse diet modification recommended by the treating team. Dysphagia, 27 (1), 81–87.

Kinder, R., 2016. An interdisciplinary approach to dysphagia. Provider – Long Term and Post-Acute Care. Available at: https://www.providermagazine.com/Monthly-Issue/2016/March/Pages/An-Interdisciplinary-Approach-To-Dysphagia.aspx. Accessed October 7, 2021.

Kjaersgaard, A., 2013. Difficulties in Swallowing and Eating Following Acquired Brain Injury – From a Professional and a Patient Perspetive. University of Southern Denmark, Hammel Neurorehabilitation and Research Centre Ph.D. Thesis.

Leopold, N.A., Kagel, M.C., 1996. Pre-pharyngeal dysphagia in Parkinson's disease. Dysphagia 11 (1), 14–122.

Logemann, J.A., 1998. Evaluation and Treatment of Swallowing Disorders. Pro-Ed, Austin, TX.

Low, J., Wyles, C., Wilkinson, T., Sainsbury, R., 2001. The effect of compliance on clinical outcomes for patients with dysphagia on videofluoroscopy. Dysphagia 16 (2), 123–127.

Mackay, L.E., Morgan, A.S., Bernstein, B.A., 1999. Factors affecting oral feeding with severe traumatic brain injury. J. Head Trauma Rehab. 14 (5), 435–447.

Matsuo, K., Hiiemae, K.M., Gonzalez-Fernandez, M., Palmer, J.B., 2008. Respiration during feeding on solid food: alterations in breathing during mastication, pharyngeal bolus aggregation, and swallowing. J. Appl. Physiol. 104, 674–681.

McCurtin, A., Healy, C., Kelly, L., Murphy, F., Ryan, J., Walsh, J., 2018. Plugging the patient evidence gap: what patients with swallowing disorders post-stroke say about thickened liquids. Int. J. Lang. Commun. Disord. 53 (1), 30–39.

McGrail, A., Kelchner, L.N., 2012. Adequate oral fluid intake in hospitalized stroke patients: does viscosity matter? Rehab. Nurs. 37 (5), 252–257.

Miller, A.J., 2008. The neurobiology of swallowing and dysphagia. Dev. Disabil. Res. Rev. 14 (2), 77–86.

Mistry, S., Hamdy, S., 2008. Neural control of feeding and swallowing. Phys. Med. Rehab. Clin. North Am. 19 (4), 709–728.

O'Keeffe, S.T., 2018. Use of modified diets to prevent aspiration in oropharyngeal dysphagia: is current practice justified? BMC Geriatr. 18 (1), 1–10.

Perry, L., Love, C.P., 2001. Screening for dysphagia and aspiration in acute stroke: a systematic review. Dysphagia, 16 (1), 7–18.

Royal College of Physicians, 2010. Oral Feeding Difficulties and Dilemmas. Royal College of Physicians. London.

Sharp, H.M., Bryant, K.N., 2003. Ethical issues in dysphagia: when patients refuse assessment or treatment. Semin. Speech Lang. 24 (4), 285–300. Copyright © 2003 by Thieme Medical Publishers Inc., 333 Seventh Avenue, New York, NY 10001m USA.

Shune, S.E., Moon, J.B., Goodman, S.S., 2016. The effects of age and pre-oral sensorimotor cues on anticipatory mouth movement during swallowing. J. Speech Lang. Hearing Res. 59 (2), 195–205.

Singh, S., 2006. Dysphagia in stroke patients. Postgrad. Med. J. 82 (968), 383–391.

Smithard, D.S., 2015. Dysphagia: prevalence, management and side effects. Nurs. Pract. 82.

Westergren, A., 2006. Detection of eating difficulties after stroke: a systematic review. Int. Nurs. Rev. 53 (2), 143–149.

Williams, V., Boyle, G., Jepson, M., Swift, P., Williamson, T., Heslop, P., 2014. Best interests decisions: professional practices in health and social care. Health Social Care Commun. 22 (1), 78–86.

Chapter 12

# Nutrition and dietetics in rehabilitation

Joanne Sim and Rachel K. Taylor

## Chapter outline

## Abstract

This chapter will provide an overview of the changing nutritional needs of patients within complex rehabilitation and the barriers and challenges in meeting the nutritional requirements of this patient group. The chapter explores how dietitians can work collaboratively with the interdisciplinary team and the benefits this brings to patients. The chapter encourages the reader to think about how the interdisciplinary team can promote nutrition as part of the rehabilitation journey. The chapter will focus on ethical and difficult decisions around nutrition in complex rehabilitation. A case study and reflective questions are presented to help consolidate learning.

A Practical Approach to Interdisciplinary Complex Rehabilitation.
DOI: https://doi.org/10.1016/B978-0-7020-8276-4.00012-6

**Keywords**
Dietitian; Nutrition; Nutritional status; Malnutrition; Nutritional support; Weight management

## Aims

1. Discuss challenges and barriers in achieving optimal nutritional status for patients requiring complex rehabilitation, and provide practical guidance on overcoming these.
2. Explore how dietitians can work within the IDT.

## Objectives

1. To understand how different stages of the rehabilitation journey can impact on nutritional requirements.
2. To explore how malnutrition can impact on recovery.
3. Discuss strategies used to help prevent and manage malnutrition.
4. Consider nutrition in relation to hydration, pressure sores, bowel habits, medication, and bone health.
5. To understand the factors that can lead to excess weight gain in the rehabilitation setting.
6. To describe strategies used to promote healthy eating habits.
7. Consider collaborative working between dietitians and the IDT.
8. Think about some ethical and difficult decisions around nutrition.

## Nutrition and dietetics in rehabilitation

Nutritional assessment and management is a key aspect of facilitating and supporting patients to achieve their maximum rehabilitation potential. Therefore the input of a specialist dietitian within a complex rehabilitation interdisciplinary team (IDT) is important. This chapter will look at the nutritional challenges faced by patients with complex rehabilitation needs.

## Nutritional aims during rehabilitation

The nutritional needs of patients in rehabilitation vary widely depending on diagnosis, comorbidities, and the stage of the rehabilitation journey (Table 12.1). Patients' nutritional goals on admission to hospital, when acutely unwell, will vary from the nutritional goals during active rehabilitation and in the community. Therefore, it is important that the patient is reviewed on a regular basis by a dietitian to ensure that nutritional goals are appropriate.

In the hyperacute phase, after trauma or injury, the body will respond by mobilising glycogen stores from the liver and breaking down lean tissue to ensure that essential systems, like the nervous and immune, have sufficient energy. This is known as catabolism. During catabolism, metabolic rate and nutritional

**TABLE 12.1 Nutritional aims during rehabilitation.**

| Stage | Nutritional aim |
|---|---|
| Hyperacute | Minimise losses of lean muscle mass, maintain hydration, and establish a route of feeding |
| Acute | Aim to meet nutritional and fluid requirements via the safest route |
| Active rehabilitation | Aim to meet nutritional and fluid requirements via the safest route. Avoiding fat mass gain and address any nutritional consequences as a result of illness/injury |
| Community/slow stream | Developing long-term nutritional strategies to optimise health |

requirements increase (Vizzini and Aranda-Michel, 2011). The nutritional aim at this stage is to minimise the rate of lean tissue loss. As the patient becomes medically stable and enters active rehabilitation, catabolism reduces and the metabolic rate starts to decrease. This is called the anabolic or recovery phase. The nutritional aim of the anabolic phase is to repair and replace muscle mass and meet new nutritional requirements. Nutritional requirements are the amount of different nutrients that the body needs at a particular time. This varies depending on age, gender, clinical presentation, medical diagnosis, and physical activity. A dietetic assessment is necessary to calculate nutritional requirements.

A consequence of not meeting nutritional requirements is malnutrition.

*'Malnutrition is a state of nutrition in which a deficiency or excess (or imbalance) of energy, protein and other nutrients causes measurable adverse effects on tissue/body form and function and clinical outcome'.*
British Association for Parental and Enteral Nutrition (2018)

For the purpose of this chapter malnutrition will relate to the deficiency of nutrition.

Risk factors for malnutrition in the community include age, multiple comorbidities, drug and alcohol abuse, social isolation, finances, limited mobility, and ability to shop and prepare meals and drinks. Once admitted to hospital the risk of malnutrition for all patients increases.

Being malnourished can affect a patient's ability to participate in, and gain from, a rehabilitation programme. Physical consequences of malnutrition include reduced muscle mass, increased risk of pressure ulcers, increased risk of falls, impaired wound healing, fatigue, and lethargy. Cognitive consequences of malnutrition can be altered mood, lethargy, depression, poor concentration, and self-neglect. Ensuring the IDT understands this link between nutrition and performance is an important part of the dietitians' role within complex rehabilitation. Dietitians may need to provide training and education sessions to the IDT about nutrition. Using case studies as examples can help put theory into context.

Of patients admitted to hospital, 25–34% were found to be malnourished (Russell and Elia, 2011). Looking at particular patient groups, 17% of patients admitted to orthopaedic wards, 20% of musculoskeletal patients and 37% of patients on care of the elderly were found to be malnourished (Russell and Elia, 2011). Wong et al. (2011) in a multicentre study found that, on admission, 44% of patients with a spinal cord injury (SCI) were at risk of malnutrition.

To help identify which patients are at risk of malnutrition, it is recommended by the National Institute for Clinical Excellence that all patients are screened on admission to hospital then weekly thereafter until discharge (NICE, 2006). It is vital that a validated screening tool, which provides guidance and an action plan, is used, for example, Malnutrition Universal Screening Tool as described by BAPEN (2016). Nursing staff have a key role in implementing screening tools and ensuring all patients are screened and referred to the dietitian if required.

Nutrition support can help in the prevention and management of malnutrition. Dietitians will assess the patient so that tailored advice can be provided. Assessment takes into account diagnosis and clinical presentation, comorbidities, anthropometrics (assessing nutritional status by external measurements, for example, mid upper arm circumference, weight) nutritional requirements and nutritional intake, medications, biochemistry, mobility, and bowel habits. Once the dietitian has assessed the patient, then the most appropriate method of nutrition support can be offered.

## Nutrition support

### Oral nutrition support

This is used as the first line approach when patients can consume sufficient nutrition orally. Oral nutrition support can be offered in two forms:

1. Food fortification (increasing the nutritional content of food) and additional nutritious snacks and drinks. Working with catering staff is vital to ensure appropriate meal and snack/ drink provision. Family members can also assist by providing additional food and drinks, as allowed by individual settings. Inpatient wards may have strict health and safety guidelines limiting the range of food bought in e.g. may not have refrigeration or heating facilities for patient's own food. Nursing staff and health care assistants (HCAs) can encourage and support meal and snack times throughout the day.
2. Prescribed nutritional supplements. These come in a variety of forms (milk- and juice-based drinks, shots, powders, puddings, and savoury soups). A dietitian is best placed to identify the most appropriate supplement.

### Enteral feeding

Enteral feeding is indicated if an individual is unable to meet their needs for nutrition, hydration, and medication orally. This may be due to dysphagia,

**TABLE 12.2** Routes of enteral feeding.

| Nasogastric feeding | | Gastrostomy feeding | |
|---|---|---|---|
| Advantages | Challenges | Advantages | Challenges |
| 1. Placed at bedside<br>2. No sedation<br>3. Short term<br>4. Easily removed<br>5. Safer access route than IV<br>6. Uses established route into the body | 1. Easily dislodged<br>2. Regular replacement required to avoid strictures and other issues<br>3. Discomfort or distress possible during placement or when in use<br>4. Positional confirmation required prior to each use<br>5. Risk of misplacement into lung<br>6. Unsightly<br>7. Fine bore tubes can block more easily with feed/medication<br>8. Takes a long time to bolus feed | 1. Can remain in place for several years if required<br>2. More discreet than NGT<br>3. Less likely to displace<br>4. Does not require position check before use<br>5. Wider tubes can provide flexibility in feeding plans<br>6. Variety of low profile, discrete tubes available<br>7. Balloon retained devices can be replaced at bedside if blocked or damaged | 1. Patient must be able to tolerate invasive placement<br>2. Placement can be distressing<br>3. More difficult to replace than NGT if problem occurs<br>4. Potential risk of buried bumper, infection, overgranulation<br>5. Procedure required for removal of tube if nontraction removable fixator<br>6. Balloon retained devices are more easily displaced |

decreased levels of consciousness, appetite, cognition, malabsorption, or an increase in nutritional requirements.

Enteral feeding options centre around two main alternatives (Table 12.2). The first option is nasogastric feeding where a small tube is passed through the nose, down the oesophagus, and into the stomach (Fig. 12.1). This is generally seen as the first line of treatment in an acute situation to allow the provision of nutrition, hydration, and medication, usually for a limited period of time. The second option is gastrostomy feeding. This is where an incision is made into the abdomen to allow a tube to be passed directly into the stomach through the abdominal wall (Fig. 12.2). This is most commonly done under endoscopic guidance; however, some patients may need radiological intervention for this procedure. During an endoscopic placement, the gastrostomy device is placed from inside the stomach to outside, normally a bumper is left in the stomach to hold the tube in place internally (Rahnemai-Azar et al., 2014). Radiological insertion is done by externally passing the device into the stomach through an incision, meaning a collapsible shaft is required, for example, a balloon retained

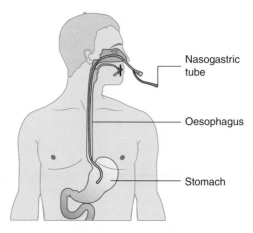

FIGURE 12.1   Nasogastric tube placement.

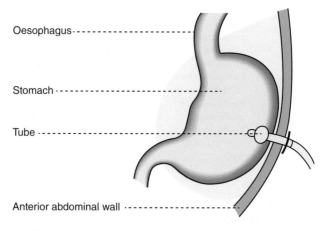

FIGURE 12.2   Gastrostomy tube placement.

gastrostomy which is inflated with sterile water once in place in the stoma tract (Shin and Park, 2010).

In some cases it may be necessary to look at post pyloric feeding (feeding directly into the jejunum) if patients suffer excessive vomiting, poor feed toler-ance or have had previous gastric surgery. This can be done via a nasojejunal tube, a standard gastrostomy with a jejunal extension, or a direct jejunostomy, depending on the circumstances and needs of the patient. This is rare in patients requiring rehabilitation.

Feeding may be by continuous infusion via an enteral feeding pump, or by several short boluses, mimicking small meals throughout the day. Modes of feeding are flexible and interchangeable whilst a patient remains in a hospital

**TABLE 12.3** Decision-making tool—bolus versus continuous feeding.

| Consideration | |
|---|---|
| Size of tube | Fine bore tubes may be difficult to bolus through |
| Ability of patient to self-administer feeds/availability of staff to assist | Bolus feeding may require administration up to eight times per day. If patient requires assistance with this, it is important to ensure this support is available from staff, family, or carers. Otherwise, continuous feeding may be advisable as it is less labour intensive |
| Symptoms: nausea, bloating, vomiting, loose bowels | Bolus feeding may present more symptoms of bloating, nausea, or vomiting therefore if a patient displays any of these symptoms, it may be advisable to use continuous feeding or convert to bolus feeding in a staged manner, being vigilant for symptoms |
| Availability of feeds in setting, viscosity, volume | High viscosity feeds may require longer to bolus therefore gravity giving sets may be advantageous, or using pump on high rate |
| Impact on rehabilitation | Continuous feeding overnight may be an option to allow freedom from pump during the day. Alternatively, bolus feeding can be scheduled around therapy and other treatment |
| Oral intake of patient | Patients' oral intake will impact on nutritional requirements from enteral nutrition. Continuous feeding may impact on the appetite and oral intake of someone who is beginning to eat, therefore minimising its impact is important. Overnight feeding or bolus feeding post meal may help |
| Fluid and medication requirements | Fluid boluses tend to be better tolerated than feed, therefore larger volumes can be used. However being mindful of the volume needed to flush medication via gastrostomy is important. Some concentrated feeds have low fluid volumes, therefore extra fluid will need to be given separately |

setting. Discussions with the IDT and patient are important to ensure the most appropriate method of feeding is implemented to allow therapy to continue safely. If the patient is taking oral diet alongside enteral nutrition, consideration of appetite, and oral feeding routines is essential to promote oral intake and minimise discomfort, without compromising nutritional intake (Table 12.3).

Towards discharge, consideration needs to be made on what fits best for the patient. Patients, family members, and carers can be trained to administer enteral feeding regimens whether continuous or bolus. If outside help is required, it is worth considering the impact on the number of care calls needed, whether this can be supported, or whether it fits with the patient's daily routines, working with the social worker and rehabilitation coordinator can help with discharge planning. Administering the feed and gastrostomy site care can be incorporated into patients' rehabilitation, if appropriate, for example, the patient can work towards gastrostomy site care with nursing staff during personal care sessions.

## Parental nutrition support

When it is not possible to provide nutrition via the oral or enteral route, patients receive all nutrition and fluids via the central or peripheral vein—this is rare in rehabilitation settings.

# Other nutritional considerations in rehabilitation

As well as malnutrition, there are other challenges in meeting patients' nutritional needs in rehabilitation. Some of these challenges are discussed below.

## Hydration

Promoting hydration, and ensuring adequate support with fluids, is key in preventing dehydration. Dehydration can be caused by a lack of fluids consumed, or excessive fluid loss, for example, through diarrhoea or excessive sweat. Patients with reduced upper limb mobility or dysphagia, who do not receive appropriate assessment and support, are at risk of not meeting their fluid requirements. As well as hands-on support to drink, patients may also need regular prompting and encouragement from all members of the IDT. Dehydration can impact negatively on cognitive function, increase risk of pressure ulcers, acute kidney injury, and physical performance in therapy sessions.

## Pressure ulcers and wound healing

Immobility, muscle wasting, devices, low body mass index (BMI), and poor nutrition are all risk factors for pressure ulcers. Patients may also present with wounds post injury or surgery. Collaborative working between the dietitian, tissue viability, and the IDT is important in the prevention and management of pressure ulcers.

## Bowel habits

Changes in bowel habits can be a result of many factors:

1. Patients experiencing prolonged periods of reduced mobility or immobilisation

**TABLE 12.4** Side effects of medication.

| Medication | Side effects |
| --- | --- |
| Long-term analgesia | Constipation |
| Anticonvulsants | Negative impact on bone mineral density |
| Muscle relaxants | Gastrointestinal disturbance |
| Neuropathic analgesia | Contribute to weight gain |

2. Reduced fluid intake
3. Changes in diet
4. Neurogenic bowel dysfunction
5. Medication, for example, long-term analgesia

If laxatives are indicated, then it is important to work collaboratively with the medical team to ensure that the most appropriate is prescribed.

## Medication

Working with the medical and nursing team is important in identifying and minimising side effects of medication on patients' nutritional status (Table 12.4).

## Bone health

Optimising bone mineral density and minimising bone loss are important in reducing the risk of fractures in patients who are at risk of falls, and helps with bone formation after fractures.

Factors that can impact on bone mineral density are:

1. A prolonged admission with limited access to outdoor space especially over the summer months which can have a negative impact on sun exposure and the resulting vitamin D synthesis
2. Lack of weight bearing exercise
3. Poor nutritional intake
4. Medication, for example, corticosteroids, anticonvulsants

## Factors affecting weight gain and strategies to improve outcomes

Entering the active rehabilitation phase of illness or injury may signify recovery; improving the wellbeing and mental health of the patient as well as increasing appetite and oral intake.

Weight changes during rehabilitation have been well documented (Crenn et al., 2013; Duraski et al., 2014). Some studies have shown that having a BMI in the overweight or obese category during rehabilitation can have a negative

**TABLE 12.5 Factors that can lead to weight gain.**

| Medical factors | Changes in metabolic rate | Medications (steroids, some anticonvulsants, antidepressant, and antipsychotic medication) can predispose to weight gain | Restricted mobility and physical activity levels leading to lower energy requirements |
|---|---|---|---|
| Patient-related factors | Increasing appetite | Mood, emotional eating, eating through boredom | Families providing 'treats', additional food |
| Catering/nutritional goals | Inappropriate prescribed nutritional supplements | Inflexible menus, catering options | Lack of dietetic cover may mean nutritional goals are not set or not appropriate for the different stages of patients rehabilitation journey |

impact on outcomes in self-care (Stenson et al., 2011), motor (Tian et al., 2013), and mobility ratings (Stenson et al., 2011). Avoiding extremes of BMI is important not only for optimising functional outcomes, but also for promoting long-term good health and minimising the development of comorbidities later in life (Dreer et al., 2018).

Unintentional weight gain during complex rehabilitation is multifactorial (Table 12.5). By developing an understanding of the challenges and barriers for this patient group, the IDT can adopt a team approach to help support individual patients.

Following an SCI, patients can experience the loss of lean body mass, resulting in a lower resting metabolic rate. A lower resting metabolic rate can mean lower daily energy expenditure and fewer calories required. If dietary intake is not corrected to meet the new lower calorie requirements, weight gain can be a consequence. There is also a danger of patients developing sarcopenic obesity as the levels of lean muscle mass decrease due to inactivity as body fat levels increase (Pelletier et al., 2016).

A systematic review and meta-analysis conducted by Farkas et al. (2018) highlighted that the problem with nutritional advice for patients with chronic SCI is that there are currently no dietary guidelines specifically for this patient group. The review found that there is excessive energy intake in the SCI population which contributes to obesity and obesity-related comorbidities including Type 2 diabetes and cardiovascular disease. The prevalence of obesity in patients with SCI found in one study was 29.9% and the percentage of people who were overweight was 65.8% (Gupta et al., 2006).

Patients who are obese when they enter rehabilitation may have worse functional outcomes for self-care and mobility and may require additional time and support with activities, for example, personal care, compared to a patient who is a healthy weight (Stenson et al., 2011).

The challenges of weight gain are not limited to patients who have reduced mobility or altered body composition. Patients with brain injuries can also be at risk of weight gain post injury (Duraski et al., 2014; Table 12.6 ).

Weight management treatment should follow an evidence-based approach. Dietary advice is generally based on the Eatwell Guide (Fig. 12.3). Many diet plans aimed at specific conditions, for example, multiple sclerosis, have been developed and publicised, however, there is little evidence to support these, and some may have detrimental consequences, therefore claims should be interpreted with caution (British Dietetic Association, 2015). Many fad and celebrity endorsed diets and meal plans are available to the public; however, there is often no, or limited, evidence to prove their efficacy or safety.

Communication of the evidence-based healthy eating guidelines can be undertaken in a variety of ways to best suit the patient, their style of learning and physical and cognitive needs. Individual support and information sharing sessions are the traditional choice of dietetic care provision; this is useful, particularly in the first instance, to assess dietary habits, beliefs, and knowledge of healthy eating and weight loss strategies. Cognitive impairment or fatigue may limit the effectiveness of intense one-to-one interview style interventions; therefore, more practical input may have more success.

Miller and Rollnick (2012) describe motivational interviewing as a 'collaborative, person-centred form of guiding to elicit and strengthen motivation to change' (p. 12). The techniques described in motivational interviewing literature encourage active listening and drawing out the patient's intrinsic motivation, by using their own ideas to elicit change. Evidence suggests that this is a more successful approach than traditional information giving sessions.

Working closely with occupational therapy to facilitate cooking sessions, either in groups or as individuals, can be valuable in demonstrating principles of healthy eating alongside improving confidence in the kitchen. Joint IDT goals looking at food shopping and meal preparation can be of value where physical and cognitive impairments are present, or where the patient's premorbid role did not particularly feature meal preparation.

Educating the IDT around healthy eating can encourage them to engage in conversations with patients regarding behaviour change and facilitate a whole team approach, this may be especially important where a patient's cognition has been impaired and the traditional 1:1 dietetic consultation is not the most effective way of communication.

Visual props, for example, fat models, portion size guides, and picture menus can aid learning and understanding, reinforcing concepts that have been taught

**TABLE 12.6 Nutritional impact of brain injury.**

| Presentation | Nutritional implications | Examples of solutions |
|---|---|---|
| Receptive aphasia | Reduced ability to read or interpret menus | 1:1 menu support, communication aids, likes/dislikes questionnaire, picture menus |
| Expressive aphasia | Reduced ability to communicate menu choices, hunger/thirst, food likes/dislikes, nausea, etc. | |
| Executive function<br><br>1. Planning<br>2. Organising<br>3. Making decisions<br>4. Behaviour control<br>5. Problem solving<br>6. Attention<br>7. Social skills<br>8. Flexible thinking<br>9. Emotional | Planning meals, preparing shopping lists, food shopping, and makingmeals<br>Antisocial behaviour at meal times<br>Hyperphagia<br>Apathy—resulting in lack of interest to pick meals from a menu, enjoyment at meal times | Working with speech and language therapy to help with communication aids. Working with occupational therapist/nursing and family to help with meal preparation, support at meal times. Working with psychology if mood and emotions are impacting on eating and drinking. A whole team approach is needed to help lessen the impact of hyperphagia on a patients' nutritional intake |
| Loss of appetite control | Hyperphagia to all food or a particular food | Support with food and drink choices, portion control and timings of meals. Looking at environment and avoid using food as reward |
| Hormonal disturbances | Constipation, weight gain | Advice on fluid and fibre to help maintain regular bowel motions<br>Healthy eating advice from a qualified professional |
| Ataxia | Difficulties with movement getting food into the mouth | Working with occupational therapy looking at techniques and equipment |

(*continued on next page*)

**TABLE 12.6** Nutritional impact of brain injury—cont'd

| Presentation | Nutritional implications | Examples of solutions |
| --- | --- | --- |
| Apraxia | Unable to select the correct piece of equipment, e.g., a fork instead of a straw | Working with occupational therapy looking at techniques and equipment |
| Hemiplegia | Ability to cut food up | Working with Occupational Therapy looking at techniques and equipment |
| Perception Spatial awareness Manipulating objects | May need assistance to cut up food, place utensil into hand and assist with placing food into mouth | Working with Occupational Therapy looking at techniques and equipment |
| Vision | Ability to be independent with preparing meals, may need assistance with placing drinks into the patients' hand and assistance with cutting up and eating | Working with occupational therapy looking at techniques and equipment. Support from staff, family, and friends |

in more formal ways. These can be used for patients and staff alike, and generate discussion around dietary habits.

## Dietetics role within the IDT

Collaborative working with other members of the IDT can be an effective use of time and resources. Joint working can emphasise the importance of nutritional goals and like a jigsaw, interconnect with other aspects of rehabilitation. It is important for members of the IDT to understand the role nutrition has within rehabilitation and how nutritional status can impact positively and negatively on a patient's rehabilitation journey. Each interaction between health professional and patient can be seen as an opportunity to empower the patient to make better choices towards shared goals. Below are some examples of how dietitians can work with members of the IDT within complex rehabilitation.

## Catering

Ensuring good links with catering is important in supporting patients meet their nutritional requirements. Inpatient catering does have its limitations: extent of the menu, meal preparation, and kitchen facilities, snack provision and special menus catering for religion, dysphagia, allergies, and ethical choices. Inpatient complex rehabilitation patients can have extended periods of admission which

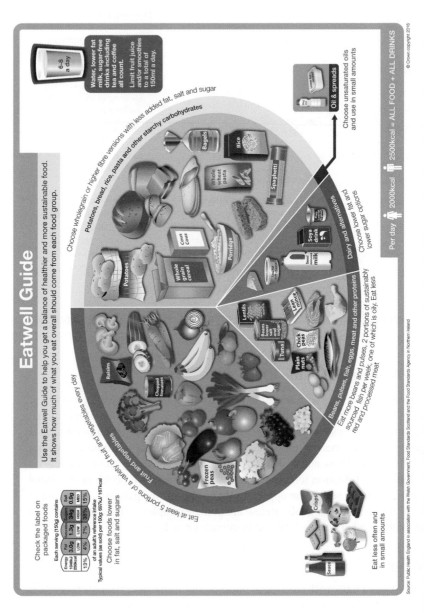

**FIGURE 12.3** Eatwell guide. From Food standards Scotland: the eatwell guide. Available at: https://www.foodstandards.gov.scot/consumers/healthy-eating/eatwell.

can result in menu fatigue. Working alongside patients, families, catering, and ward managers to see if there is opportunity for food and drinks to be bought in to a setting to help increase variety or if catering can offer alternative meals/snacks, etc. Negotiating flexibility to use staff canteen facilitates or arranging special menus for occassions, holidays, etc. can help to improve issues like menu fatigue.

## Nursing and health care assistants

Nursing and HCAs are important members of the IDT in supporting patients nutritionally. They can identify patients who are at risk of malnutrition, monitor tolerance to artificial feeding and oral supplements, support at meal times, monitor bowel habits and fluid intake. A close working relationship is vital between the dietitian, nursing, and HCAs to optimise patients' nutritional status.

## Occupational therapy

The meal time experience encompasses a wide range of points all of which can have an impact on the patient nutritionally. For example, ensuring all toileting needs are met premeal, correct seating, and table setup, distractions are identified and limited and support is provided if required for feeding. Ensuring a positive meal time experience will give the patient the best chance to enjoy the food they have ordered and help achieve their nutritional requirements. Working with occupational therapy along with nursing staff is vital to ensure this is achieved.

Impaired executive function can affect a wide variety of day-to-day tasks like meal planning and maintaining healthy eating habits. Dietitians and occupational therapists can work collaboratively to incorporate nutritional goals into therapy, for example, joining up patients' healthy eating goals into a meal preparation task.

## Physiotherapy

Physiotherapy sessions can be negatively impacted on by many factors, some already discussed in the chapter, for example, dehydration and malnutrition. It is important that physiotherapists and dietitians communicate their own professional goals to ensure a collaborative approach. For example, timings of enteral feeding regimens and physiotherapy sessions can be coordinated to ensure patient safety.

## Psychology

Emotional eating can be a result of many factors in rehabilitation. A coping strategy or low mood can influence food choices; this may result in weight gain or weight loss which ultimately can have short- and long-term implications for rehabilitation potential and health. By working together dietetics and psychology can identify patients at risk and help facilitate strategies to limit the impact of emotional eating.

## Speech and language therapist

Any impairment of communication can impact on a patient nutritionally. Receptive/expressive aphasia may impact on the patient's ability to read a menu, order meals, request a drink, etc. Working closely with speech and language therapy is vital to ensure the most effective way of communication is used.

If the patient has dysphagia then they may be placed on altered textured meals or drinks. It is important dietitians, speech and language therapist, catering, and nursing all work together to ensure the appropriate menus are provided, there is support at meal times and staff are appropriately trained to maintain patient safety, for example, a red tray system, correct signage.

## Therapy assistants

Patients with either cognitive or physical impairments may mean they are unable to independently choose from the menu or communicate their likes/dislikes, ask for additional snacks and drinks and could be at risk of not meeting their nutritional requirements. Therapy assistants are able to provide this 1:1 support, using picture menus, liaising with family members, providing likes and dislikes questionnaires, spending time supporting the patient with taking additional snacks.

## Medical team

Patients who are struggling with common symptoms and medication side effects, e.g. constipation, diarrhoea, nausea and vomiting, can be effectively managed through working together with medics. Managing biochemistry, common long-term conditions like diabetes, and addressing feeding issues including the planning and management of enteral feeds also benefit from joint working.

## Ethical/difficult decisions about nutrition

Along the rehabilitation journey there are lots of challenges to meeting nutritional goals, therefore it is vital dietetics work alongside the IDT and patient to improve outcomes.

The principles of ethics (Summer, 2014) apply as much to the area of patient nutrition as they do to any other aspect of patient care. To highlight some of the difficult situations and decisions that may arise around the subject of nutrition, the following short case studies are designed to provoke thought and reflection. They are not intended to provide direction for a particular situation. All situations need to be evaluated individually.

### Example 1: Nil by mouth (NBM) and the need for artificial nutrition support

Your patient has an unsafe swallow, recommended to remain nil by mouth. They have fluctuating levels of consciousness and therefore unable to consent to the insertion of a nasogastric feeding tube. Their family have been involved in discussions and are concerned about him becoming weaker if he does not receive nutrition therefore they agree that feeding is a priority. However the patient continues to be agitated and has pulled out several NG tubes before any feed or medication could be given via this route.

Things to consider:

1. If the patient's levels of alertness are fluctuating, take this into account when discussing feeding tubes and insertion. Are you able to ascertain any reasons for the tubes being pulled out?
2. Is the patient pulling out other supportive devices, for example, catheter, IV fluids, etc. If isolated to feeding tubes, consider if this is a method of the patient communicating their wishes.
3. What are the findings from speech therapy assessments? Can they give an indication of prognosis of swallow? Could it recover quickly, or is long-term feeding indicated?
4. If long-term feeding is indicated, it may be worth considering a gastrostomy tube insertion. Consider waiting times for the procedure – can you wait, or does an interim measure need to be considered.
5. What is the least restrictive option for intervention in the patient's best interest?
6. Consider providing 1:1 support for the patient to help settle the agitation and help prevent the nasogastric tube being displaced.
7. Consider nasal bridle (a retention device) to discourage patient from pulling on NG tube.
8. Consider use of mitts or restraint to prevent pulling of NG tube.
9. Bear in mind any intervention in the best interests of the patient should be the least restrictive option wherever possible.
10. Ask for support from a nutrition team if available locally.

## Example 2: Family and team disagree

Your patient has severe dysphagia, nil by mouth and receives all nutrition via gastrostomy tube. The patient does not have capacity to make a decision regarding method of feeding. The family feels that the patient's quality of life is poor and that his premorbid wish would have been not to be artificially fed, even given the ultimate consequence being death.

Things to consider:

1. Team involvement in determining what the patient's potential for recovery is, physically, cognitively, and with swallowing.
2. Consider length of time from injury and whether decision making should allow more time for recovery.

3. Is there an alternative to strict NBM? Could oral trials/sips of water, etc. be offered to improve quality of life, either safely, or with all parties agreeing to accept the risk?
4. Gather information of premorbid attitude to risk, information from patient, family and friends, advanced directives.
5. If fluctuating capacity, choose times when alertness and capacity are at their best, even if the patient does not pass a capacity assessment, it may aid information gathering.
6. Be mindful of a change in attitude, survival instinct and subjective nature of interpreting someone else's quality of life. For example, the patient being able to watch his children play may be enough motivation for him to want to survive, even if he is unable to join in with the play.
7. Ultimately, the treating team needs to make a best interests decision, on whether the patient's feeding should be discontinued. This should include feedback from the patient, friends, and family; however, the team has the overarching responsibility for the best interests of the patient. Decisions around withdrawal or withholding of nutrition do not necessarily need to go to court, if all parties agree with the decision made in best interests. If there is disagreement, the team may need to go through mediation or court for an overarching decision to be made.
8. If a decision is made to withdraw enteral feeding, a second decision needs to be made around whether it is acceptable to allow oral intake, taking into account the implications on patient safety balanced with quality of life (Royal College of Physicians and British Society of Gastroenterology, 2010).

## Example 3: Excessive weight gain

Your patient has gained excessive weight since admission to the rehabilitation unit following a head injury. Their VP shunt has become obstructed on more than one occasion. The neurosurgeon believes this is due to increased fat mass. The patient has also developed impaired glucose tolerance. He has a cognitive impairment which means he can forget he has eaten at times and also presents with excessive appetite or disinhibition around food. Some aggressive behaviour has been shown when denied food. A capacity assessment has shown that the patient lacks capacity around the risk of further weight gain on his health.

Things to consider:

1. Does the patient have any awareness or thoughts around weight gain? Does he understand the implications of further weight gain?
2. What was his premorbid attitude to weight/body image/fitness?
3. Is there a pattern to overeating?
4. What are his food sources? Family bringing in food, takeaways being brought in by family and friends? Staff providing extra sandwiches and meals?

5. Are family and friends on board with need to address weight?
6. Is it appropriate to limit food intake? Does this have implications for staff providing food—nursing staff, ward caterers, visitors?
7. External input to halt weight gain is likely needed in this case, as the patient lacks awareness of the health implications. This will require a whole team approach from dietetics, therapy, psychology, medical, and nursing staff, as well as catering staff and visitors, if it is to be successful. Managing the patient's behaviour if not being provided with what he asks may be a challenge for staff, and may require support and strategies to be put in place.

## Summary

Nutritional requirements of patients vary greatly throughout the rehabilitation journey from acute through to community. It is important that dietitians are part of the IDT to facilitate ongoing nutritional assessments and to ensure nutritional goals are appropriate. It is essential for the IDT to have an understanding of the role a dietitian has within complex rehabilitation and how the patient can benefit from joint working.

### Reflective questions

Ben is a 60-year-old gentleman who was admitted with polytrauma following a car versus motorbike road traffic accident. He sustained a traumatic brain injury, below knee amputation and C2 spinal fracture with halo fixator in situ. Bilateral cerebellar and occipital infarcts: cortical blindness post injury. Ben had a long stay on ITU followed by an admission to a hyper acute level 1 rehab ward, 47 days post injury.

On initial dietetic assessment, he was strictly nil by mouth and had lost 12.5% of his body weight since admission (clinically significant).

- What route of feeding would you consider for Ben?

Ben progressed well in Level 1 rehab. He began using a prosthetic limb in therapy and commenced oral trials of modified texture with speech and language therapists. He had a radiologically inserted gastrostomy tube in situ, providing all his nutritional, hydration, and medication needs. He was transferred to Level 2 active rehabilitation where his swallow progressed quickly to allow him more variety in his diet.

- What barriers could prevent Ben achieving a good nutritional intake?
- What support could the treating team put in place to help overcome some of these barriers?
- Can you foresee any issues with Ben's long-term nutritional management?

# References

British Association for Parental and Enteral Nutrition. (2016) Introducing MUST British Artificial and Parental and Enteral Nutrition. Available at: https://www.bapen.org.uk/screening-and-must/must/introducing-must. Accessed September 15, 2019.

British Association for Parental and Enteral Nutrition. (2018) Introduction to Malnutrition. Available at: https://www.bapen.org.uk/malnutrition-undernutrition/introduction-to-malnutrition. Accessed October 3, 2019.

British Dietetic Association (2015) Policy statement: the use of alternative diets and supplementation in the management of multiple sclerosis. Available at: https://www.bda.uk.com/improvinghealth/healthprofessionals/policy_statements/ms_management. Accessed October 10, 2019.

Crenn, P., Hamchaoui, S., Bourget-Massari, A., Hanachi, M., Melchoir, J.C., Azouvi, P, 2013. Changes in weight after traumatic brain injury in adult patients: a longitudinal study. Clin. Nutr. 33, 348–353.

Dreer, L.E., Ketchum, J.M., Novack, A.T., Bogner, J., Felix, E., Corrigan, J.D., Johnson Greene, D., Hammond, F.M., 2018. Obesity and overweight problems among individuals 1 to 25 years following brain injury: a NIDILRR traumatic brain injury model systems study. J. Head Trauma Rehab. 33, 246–256.

Duraski, S.A., Lovell, L., Roth, B.S., Roth, E., 2014. Nutritional intake, body mass index, and activity in postacute traumatic brain injury: a preliminary study. Rehab. Nurs. 39, 140–146.

Farkas, G.J., Pitot, A., Berg, A.S., Gater, D.G., 2018. Nutritional status in chronic spinal cord injury: a systematic review and meta-analysis. Spinal Cord 57, 3–17.

Gupta, N., White, K.T., Sandford, P.R., 2006. Body mass index in spinal cord injury – a retrospective study. Spinal Cord 44, 92–94.

Miller, W., Rollnick, S., 2012. Motivational Interviewing: Helping People Change, third ed. Guilford Press, New York.

National Institute for Clinical Excellence Clinical Guideline (CG32), 2006. Nutrition Support for Adults: Oral Nutrition Support, Enteral Tube Feeding and Parental Nutrition. Available at: https://www.nice.org.uk/guidance/CG32.

Pelletier, C.A., Miyatani, M., Giangregorio, L., Craven, B.C., 2016. Sarcopenic obesity in adults with spinal cord injury: a cross sectional study. Arch. Phys. Med. Rehab. 97, 1931–1937.

Rahnemai-Azar, A.A., Rahnemaiazar, A.A., Naghshizadian, R., Kurtz, A., Farkas, D.T., 2014. Percutaneous endoscopic gastrostomy: indications, technique, complications and management. World J. Gastroenterol. 20 (24), 7739–7751. doi:10.3748/wjg.v20.i24.7739. Available at: https://www.wjgnet.com/1007-9327/full/v20/i24/7739.htm. Accessed September 7, 2019.

Royal College of Physicians and British Society of Gastroenterology, 2010. Oral Feeding Difficulties and Dilemmas: A Guide to Practical Care, Particularly Towards the End of Life. Royal College of Physicians, London. Available at: https://www.rcplondon.ac.uk/projects/outputs/oral-feeding-difficulties-and-dilemmas.

Russell, C.A., Elia, M. (2011) Nutrition Screening Surveys in Hospitals in the UK 2007-2011. British Artificial and Parental and Enteral Nutrition. Available at: https://www.bapen.org.uk/pdfs/nsw/bapen-nsw-uk.pdf. Accessed September 27, 2019.

Shin, J.H., Park, A.W., 2010. Updates on percutaneous radiologic gastrostomy/gastrojejunostomy and jejunostomy. Gut Liver 4 (Suppl. 1), S25–S31. doi:10.5009/gnl.2010.4.S1.S25. Available at: https://www.gutnliver.org/journal/view.html?doi=10.5009/gnl.2010.4.S1.S25. Accessed September 4, 2019.

Stenson, K.W., Deutsch, A.M.D., Heinemann, A.W., Chen, D., 2011. Obesity and inpatient rehabilitation outcomes for patients with a traumatic spinal cord injury. Arch. Phys. Med. Rehab. 92, 384–390.

Summer, J., 2014. Principles of healthcare ethics. In: Morrison, E.E., Furlong, B. (Eds.), Health Care Ethics: Critical Issues for the 21st Century. Jones & Bartlett Learning, Burlington, pp. 47–50.

Tian, W., Hsieh, C.H., Dejong, G., Backus, D., Groah, S., Ballard, P.H., 2013. Role of body weight in therapy participation and rehabilitation outcomes among individuals with traumatic spinal cord injury. Arch. Phys. Med. Rehab. 94, s125–s136.

Vizzini, A., Aranda-Michel, J., 2011. Nutritional support in head injury. Nutrition 27 (2), 129–132. Available at: http://dx.doi.org/10.1016/j.nut.2010.05.004. Accessed July 13, 2019.

Wong, S.S., Derry, F., Harini, S., Grimble, G., Forbes, A., 2011. Validation of the spinal nutrition screening tool (SNST) in patients with spinal cord injuries (SCI): result from a multicentre study. Eur. J. Clin. Nutr. 66, 382–387. Available at: https://www.nature.com/articles/ejcn2011209. Accessed November 2, 2019.

Chapter 13

# Early vocational rehabilitation within an interdisciplinary context

Ray Langford

## Chapter outline

**Abstract**

This chapter will describe the role that the field of vocational rehabilitation can play in the overall management of individuals with complex rehabilitation needs, both within the context of the interdisciplinary healthcare team but also in the wider local business and education communities.

Whilst the centrality of work and education in everyday life is hard to overlook, individuals with complex rehabilitation needs face daunting challenges in returning to work and education. These challenges can include significant, temporary or permanent functional capacity, and difficulties in personal adjustment. In addition, if the individual desires to return to work or education, they are required to navigate around disclosure, concerns about their fitness to work or study, and how they might negotiate support from their employer or educational establishment.

This chapter seeks to demonstrate that by embedding the practice of vocational rehabilitation into the interdisciplinary context, it can make a contribution not only to the successful return to employment and education but also to better overall outcomes for the individual.

The chapter considers: the models of service delivery; how vocational rehabilitation practice can be embedded into the interdisciplinary team context; what is meant by specialist vocational rehabilitation; and how to make vocational rehabilitation person-centred and the interventions used in its delivery.

A Practical Approach to Interdisciplinary Complex Rehabilitation.
DOI: https://doi.org/10.1016/B978-0-7020-8276-4.00013-8

**222**

**Keywords**
Vocational rehabilitation; Employment; Education; Interdisciplinary context; Traumatic injury; Sickness absence; Vocational case management; Career redirection; Vocational assessment; Fitness for work

## Aim

To assist the reader in understanding the role that vocational rehabilitation plays in the interdisciplinary team (IDT) management of patients with complex rehabilitation needs.

## Objectives

1. To introduce the reader to the practice of vocational rehabilitation within the United Kingdom.
2. To introduce the three-level model of vocational rehabilitation.
3. To illustrate how vocational rehabilitation is embedded into interdisciplinary working.
4. To focus on specialist vocational rehabilitation.
5. To identify how the principles of patient-centred care are applied in vocational rehabilitation.
6. To describe the vocational assessments and interventions that are commonly provided.
7. To describe the interface between health care and the workplace/education environment.

## Introduction

Vocational rehabilitation is the process that enables those who have suffered a traumatic injury or illness to be supported to return to (or remain in) employment or education. Its focus is to help people to retain or regain the ability to work, rather than to treat the illness or injury. This process draws from a wide range of services, assessments, and interventions.

This chapter will explore how vocational rehabilitation can be provided within the context of an IDT, working with patients who have complex rehabilitation needs. It will illustrate how early vocational rehabilitation can both complement and inform the core provision of complex rehabilitation, and enhance both the vocational, and overall, patient rehabilitation outcomes. The national service framework for long-term neurological conditions (DH Long-term Conditions NSF Team, 2005) and the BSRM Guidelines on Assessment and Rehabilitation for People with Long Term Neurological Conditions (British Society of Rehabilitation Medicine, 2010) have both highlighted the need for vocational rehabilitation. However, the provision of vocational rehabilitation continues to vary across the United Kingdom.

Playford et al. (2011) led a 2-year research project which focused on the mapping of vocational rehabilitation services for people with long-term neurological conditions. The conclusion of this study was that overall, UK vocational rehabilitation services did not meet the needs of people with long-term neurological conditions, and were under-resourced in terms of staff numbers, range of disciplines, and expertise. The study also concluded that there was no consensus on how the outcome data should be collated for vocational rehabilitation, and on many occasions, it was not collated at all. The study did however find that the key mechanisms for the successful implementation of vocational rehabilitation included the presence of IDTs, and the co-location of health services with employment services.

In addition to establishing the provision of vocational rehabilitation within complex rehabilitation, it is important to understand the models that support its practice, how teams/services can successfully integrate vocational rehabilitation into standard practice, and who is required to deliver it.

## Models of service delivery

Beyond the complex rehabilitation IDT already described in this publication, there are a large array of support services helping individuals return to and remain in employment, education, and training. It is therefore important that we first understand where the approaches and interventions, provided by the IDT, fit into this broader context. This book has already supported the provision of timely rehabilitation following traumatic injury or illness, demonstrating the importance of team working, communication, and shared interdisciplinary rehabilitation goals. There is a growing recognition that return to work/education is a process which the individual prepares for, and different patients have differing needs. The IDT can therefore play a key role in vocational rehabilitation from the very beginning of the patient's rehabilitation pathway, engaging the patient in discussions about their vocational goals, supporting them with activities/hobbies and positive routines, and helping them to connect with others. Further specialist vocational rehabilitation assessment can help to identify any barriers the individual faces in achieving their vocational goals, assess specific individual needs to provide tailored support, and provide effective liaison between patients and relevant agencies such as other health care professionals, employers, human resource departments, occupational health services, and voluntary organisations.

The interventions described in this chapter are best described as 'early specialist vocational rehabilitation'. The exact configuration of a model for vocational rehabilitation will need to be designed around local service needs. However, the model should be comprehensive and able to support patients with information and self-management, as well as able to provide structured vocational rehabilitation interventions to support those with more complex

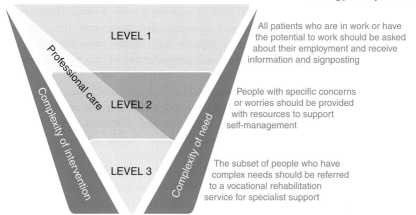

Thinking positively about work

LEVEL 1 — All patients who are in work or have the potential to work should be asked about their employment and receive information and signposting

LEVEL 2 — People with specific concerns or worries should be provided with resources to support self-management

LEVEL 3 — The subset of people who have complex needs should be referred to a vocational rehabilitation service for specialist support

FIGURE 13.1    The three-level model of work support interventions for people with cancer.

vocational needs. The model must also be agile enough to allow services to support patients at any point of their rehabilitation pathway; from acute inpatient admission to postdischarge and community settings.

One such model of delivery was set up by the National Cancer Survivorship Initiative, Work and Finance Workstream (Gail, 2012). This model is known as the Three-Level Model of Work Support for People with Cancer. Although it was originally designed for a different patient group/case mix to the one discussed here, it is also a good fit for patients with complex rehabilitation needs. Both patient groups follow a protracted period of recovery that can be multidimensional in nature, and both require well-planned support to facilitate a sustainable return to work, education, or training. The Three-Level Model enables the provision of vocational rehabilitation to be centred on patient need at any point during their recovery and values the efforts of the IDT in achieving the patient's vocational goals.

Fig. 13.1 illustrates the three distinct levels of intervention. It is important to recognise that patients may not require vocational input at each of the three levels, nor will they necessarily move through the levels in sequence. For patients affected by traumatic illness or injury, work support and vocational rehabilitation can be provided at three levels:

1. At Level 1, all of the patient's vocational needs can be supported through information and signposting. The initial process will include a screening of their previous vocational status and the identification of new needs, secondary to their illness/injury. This initial screen may immediately highlight an action that needs to be addressed, for example, signposting the patient or their advocate to an appropriate agency.

2. At Level 2 patients may have specific concerns or worries about their employment/education which could be addressed in the formulation of their rehabilitation goals and supported through self-management. It is possible that at this stage, strategies and support may involve drawing on work-specific situations. Simulations of work-related activities may be appropriate, but without the pressure of performance expectation.

3. At Level 3, the complexity of vocational need increases to require structured interventions beyond the skills and knowledge of a therapist, nurse, medic, or rehabilitation coordinator, and which are best delivered by a specialist vocational rehabilitation practitioner. At Level 3, the enhanced skill set equips the practitioner to step outside the boundaries of core health care, and into local business, charitable, and educational sectors. The focus here is on understanding the demands relating to work role or type of education to help the patient with planning a return. This enhanced skill set is likely to require additional training (beyond generic IDT working) to meet its complexity.

## Embedding vocational rehabilitation practice into the interdisciplinary team

Kärrholm et al. (2006) found that multiprofessional, coordinated rehabilitation interventions, enabled people to return to work sooner, and improved their physical, social, and emotional functioning and wellbeing. Traditionally, vocational rehabilitation was separate to the core practice of rehabilitation, and vocational needs were often only addressed at the point of discharge, primarily involving a referral to an external agency. However, by embedding vocational rehabilitation within the rehabilitation pathway, it means that there is a greater chance that these needs will be successfully met at the most appropriate time for the patient.

With early intervention, the IDT can provide advice and support to the patient, family members, and other service providers involved in the patient's care, avoiding premature decisions being made about work or education. It is essential to recognise that many patients will have already formulated beliefs about their ability to return to previous vocational roles. Therefore, the IDT should be alerted to these beliefs, as they can have a major implication, not only on the achievement of vocational outcomes, but also on general recovery and rehabilitation as a whole.

For patients affected by traumatic injury or illness there can be anxieties about their future career prospects. Such anxieties can arise at any time, thus requiring support to be available throughout a patient's rehabilitation pathway. The IDTs are best placed to provide this Level 1/2 support, as they will have formed a rapport with the patient and will have an understanding of their status and prognosis in both medical and functional terms.

If the patient triggers early for a Level 3 intervention, working alongside a vocational rehabilitation specialist will provide the IDT with a greater insight into a patient's employment and/or education roles. Specialist assessment can enhance a team's understanding of vocational needs, and tailor the patient's individual rehabilitation goals. However, care must be taken to not impose a vocational intervention too soon for the reasons outlined above.

## Specialist vocational rehabilitation

Radford et al. (2013) found that specialist vocational rehabilitation enabled more participants to return to work following a traumatic brain injury than those who were not in receipt of such specialist intervention. Significantly, they found that patients with more complex disabilities/injuries benefited more from such interventions than those with less complex disabilities/injuries.

As we have previously explored, the Three-Level Model can be used in the context of complex rehabilitation following traumatic injury or illness. This highlights the need for a specialist practitioner, with an enhanced skill set, who can deliver complex vocational interventions, work as part of the rehabilitation IDT and take on a leadership role in the management of vocational needs. This view is echoed in the Multidisciplinary Association for Spinal Cord Injury Professionals Guidelines for Vocational Rehabilitation (Multidisciplinary Association for Spinal Cord Injury Professionals, 2017).

Specialist vocational rehabilitation is unregulated in the United Kingdom and therefore not treated as a profession with specific entry requirements to practice. Most professionals delivering vocational rehabilitation do this as an extension of their core role and may struggle to find the educational opportunities to support further development of skills as a specialist vocational rehabilitation practitioner. When recruiting a specialist vocational rehabilitation practitioner, employers must consider how they will train, and retain, professionals with the required skill set. In comparison, the traditional path in the United States and Canada is to complete a bachelor's degree in a rehabilitation profession, and then to progress to earn a master's degree in vocational rehabilitation. In the 2016 document 'Planning the future: implications for occupational health; delivery and training', The Council for Work and Health (representing the Vocational Rehabilitation Association UK) published recommendations for standards, a code of practice and scope of practice, which aimed to guide the formulation of competencies required to practice as a specialist vocational rehabilitation practitioner (Council for Work and Health, 2016). Whilst this association is primarily aimed at the occupational health sector, many of the skills are transferable into the field of complex vocational rehabilitation following traumatic illness or injury. The guidelines also identified that nationally recognised multidisciplinary training in vocational rehabilitation should be made available for health professionals. Given the additional skill set that is required to deliver vocational rehabilitation at Level 3 (which will be discussed below), developing the specialist practitioner with an additional postgraduate qualification, like those undertaken by nurses working in occupational health, may have significant advantages.

To successfully incorporate and embed vocational rehabilitation specialists into the IDT, they need to work within existing rehabilitation structures and systems, including interdisciplinary meetings, goal planning, patient and family education, discharge planning, outpatient support and referrals to other agencies and peer support organisations.

## Providing patient-centred vocational rehabilitation

Picker (Davis et al., 2005), a leading International Healthcare Charity, identified the eight principles of patient-centred care conducive to a positive patient experience. Patient-centred care describes the well-established practice of caring for patients (and their families) in ways that are meaningful and valuable to the individual patient, and includes listening to, informing and involving patients in their care. It involves sharing power and responsibility and taking a holistic approach to care and needs assessment.

NHS England, in its Commissioning Guidance for Rehabilitation (NHS England, 2016), highlighted the need for people-centred services that provide good rehabilitation. It encourages commissioned services to be driven by the rehabilitation goals that are set by the people who are treated, which are centred on their needs, not their diagnosis. It also highlights the need to integrate specialist services into interdisciplinary working, and most significantly, it encourages providers to include vocational outcomes which contribute to instilling hope.

Throughout vocational rehabilitation assessment and intervention, patients should be actively involved in their goals, and their vocational needs should be addressed in a way that reflects their own unique values, preferences, and expressed needs. Taking time to address patient's vocational queries and concerns may help to identify issues that would otherwise compound the patient's sense of vulnerability and powerlessness in the face of illness and injury. Delivering vocational rehabilitation throughout the rehabilitation pathway, at different stages of a patient's recovery, increases the number of opportunities to alleviate stress and worries associated with patient vocation.

Vocational rehabilitation can help patients to understand how their impairments will impact on their life prospects, and how they might mitigate that impact through their own actions and support provided by the treating rehabilitation team. This provision of patient education aims to facilitate autonomy, self-care, and health promotion. A sense of progress and understanding of prognosis can be engendered by appropriately focusing on vocational goals well ahead of an actual return to work/education. This often requires considerable negotiation for patients to understand its relevance to them at that specific time of their recovery.

In addition to the patient themselves, the focus of specialist vocational rehabilitation intervention is on the patient's working or educational environment. This involves a thorough understanding of the demands of the role, what equipment may need providing, and carefully thought-out reasonable adjustments. By addressing the environment, barriers to a return to work/education can be removed or reduced, and patient comfort on returning can be optimised.

We have already established in previous chapters that the fear and anxiety associated with illness (adjustment to illness and the potential impact on mental health) can be as debilitating as the physical effects. Common amongst these anxieties are the impact of the illness on an individual's vocational status, prospects, and financial independence. Addressing the fears and anxieties through vocational rehabilitation practices can lead to an increased sense of wellbeing and positivity.

The involvement of family and friends is a key component of patient-centred care and is also significant in vocational rehabilitation. By involving family and friends, with the patient's permission, a more detailed assessment can be undertaken, vocational plans can be explored more comprehensively, and patients can seek reinforcement and reassurance from their trusted loved ones. Providing vocational rehabilitation throughout the patient's rehabilitation pathway ensures that vocational needs do not get lost in the transition between services and teams.

Because vocational rehabilitation is patient-centred, it is not driven by employer/organisational priorities. If returning to a former role is not realistic or desirable, then it is possible to support the patient into new pursuits that can accommodate their residual impairments. This is a key difference from the interventions offered by occupational health professionals whose involvement is conditional to the patient's continued employment and ends once the patient leaves an organisation.

## Vocational rehabilitation interventions

To this point we have considered the present status of vocational rehabilitation practice in the United Kingdom, a potential model of service delivery, how vocational rehabilitation can be embedded into interdisciplinary practice, the role of a specialist practitioner, and how the delivery of vocational intervention must be patient-centred. This next section will describe some of the interventions a specialist practitioner can provide.

1. *Vocational case management*

This is the process whereby the efforts of the IDT are managed in vocational terms to address the patients' employment/education needs or challenges. This is ideally carried out by the specialist vocational rehabilitation practitioner. These vocational needs can be either highlighted at point of referral, or emerge during the interdisciplinary assessment, given that referrals may not specifically address vocational needs. The specialist vocational rehabilitation practitioner will determine the optimum time to engage with a patient, and support colleagues to tailor their therapeutic interventions to meet specific vocational goals.

Whilst the broad goals of rehabilitation may be collaboratively determined at the point of referral, there is often a great deal of variability in the willingness of the individual patient to engage in vocational rehabilitation. This often depends on where a patient's vocational goals rank amidst their list of personal priorities. Therefore, the delivery of vocational rehabilitation interventions must reflect this variability and provide an agile patient-centred response to ensure vocational rehabilitation is meaningful. Sometimes this willingness to engage is driven by external events, such as an employer establishing contact as part of the sickness absence process, or an educator establishing the patient's future needs for support. Therefore, a frequent review of vocational needs and goals is likely to be required by the IDT, rather than a one-off consideration at the point of referral or initial assessment/goal setting.

## 2. *Vocational needs assessment*

The vocational needs assessment should be undertaken at a point in the patient's rehabilitation where it is possible to gain a full picture of their presenting situation, including symptoms, treatments, their physical, cognitive, and mental functioning, and prognosis for further recovery. The impact of these factors on their vocational goals can then be considered, together with any psychosocial strengths, challenges, and barriers to returning to work/education.

As the patient is unlikely to be ready to return to work or education at the time of referral, the assessment may identify an intervention, preparation, or the assistance required to support the individual to return in the future. Indeed, part of the assessment might be to ascertain whether they are ready to engage in vocational rehabilitation if this appears ambiguous. The conclusion of this assessment may include a vocational action plan, which requires the individual to identify goals, and steps to achieve their goals, providing the basis for rehabilitation and vocational case management.

## 3. *Job demands analysis*

An essential part of any successful vocational intervention is for all parties to have a thorough understanding of the environment in which the patient works or studies, the demands placed on the individual, and a description of the tasks involved. The world of work and education are enormously variable and require careful assessment if plans are to be realistic and achievable.

The job demands analysis is achieved through a variety of methods including, patient history taking, questionnaire completion, internet research, employer liaison, and where necessary a worksite visit. Whilst the coordination of the analysis remains the responsibility of the vocational rehabilitation specialist practitioner, the involvement of others, especially the patient, fosters a sense of collaboration which is important in ultimately achieving vocational goals.

This activity is more than just an administrative task. The analysis is about breaking down job functions into constituent parts, which enables a problem-solving approach to be used, and goals to be identified. It also makes it easier to gain an appreciation of what the job role involves, as well as making it simpler to identify reasonable adjustments.

If shared with employers, the job demands analysis can demonstrate that care and attention is being given to the establishment of realistic and achievable goals and increases the chances that they will support the process. Employers' representatives may include line or senior managers, human resource professionals, occupational health staff, and staff side representatives. At this point, the specialist vocational rehabilitation practitioner forms a broader IDT, focused on a patient's safe, successful, and sustainable return to work or study. Throughout this process, the specialist practitioner remains focused on the needs of the patient, not the organisation, and can advocate on their behalf.

### 4. Reporting on fitness for work and ability to return to education

The traditional method for a patient to obtain opinion on fitness for work is via their GP, consultant, or occupational health practitioner. However, with patients engaged in complex rehabilitation, the IDTs are in a prime position to comment on the contemporary and evolving functional status of the patient and their fitness for work/education. This can be further enhanced when those involved in rehabilitation have access to a functional job analysis and can reconcile this against the patient's functional status. Whilst several members of the IDT can report on aspects of fitness for work, the specialist vocational rehabilitation practitioner, providing Level 3 vocational rehabilitation, will be in the best position to represent the IDT with an opinion on fitness for work.

For this purpose, the Allied Health Professions Federation (2019) developed the Allied Health Professions Health and Work Report. This report is in a blank editable PDF format and is designed to clearly illustrate the patient's presenting problems, what solutions can be seen, and a summary of the patient's status. It then provides an opinion of fitness for work and whether this is conditional on workplace adjustments. The completed report is given to the patient and they are advised to share it with their employer and their GP if they feel it accurately reflects their situation.

### 5. Career redirection and vocational assessment

These interventions are aimed at patients who are unable to return to work in their previous role with or without modified duties. Without an intervention, many of these patients would fall into joblessness. Engaging the patient in a career redirection intervention, whilst they are still being seen by the IDT, can help to provide a focus on new goals that reflect their changed functional status and vocational wishes. The patient may wish to explore alternative paid employment, voluntary work, or educational opportunities. Once goals have been identified, they can work towards them with the rehabilitation IDT, supporting with patient mental health, identity, role change, and adjustment.

Vocational assessment is of key importance in career redirection. It evaluates how the patient's present functional status can be reconciled with their interests, values, transferrable skills, and qualifications. This assessment is collated, interpreted, and recorded in a document called the vocational profile.

At the point of discharge from vocational rehabilitation, the patient can be signposted to the relevant mainstream employment/educational agencies or take forward the new direction independently. Discharged patients are thus armed with the contents of the vocational profile, a set of newly identified vocational goals, a summary of their progress in rehabilitation, and their present functional status.

**6.** *The withdrawal from work on health grounds*

The withdrawal from work on health grounds may be the only possible outcome for some individuals. For those who are members of a pension scheme or have paid for income protection insurance, they may have at least some protection from financial hardship. Both the outcome and the process can be challenging for the patient and their family.

Specialist vocational rehabilitation can focus on helping the patient to navigate their way through the formal process of ill health retirement and supporting the patient to address what life might look like once they have withdrawn from work on health grounds. This intervention can therefore have a major bearing on their longer-term personal adjustment and mental wellbeing.

**7.** *Support with education and training*

For many patients who are receiving complex rehabilitation, further education is a key vocational goal, and vocational rehabilitation can play a central role in enabling this goal to become reality. Many will want to continue with the studies that they have already started, whilst others will see education as a new goal to be pursued, either as part of retraining for alternative employment, or as a replacement for formalised work. Much like work, accessing education can be problematic following illness and injury and require further specialist intervention. This might involve direct liaison with the education provider or supporting students with their application for disabled student allowance.

**8.** *Case coordination/clinical leadership*

Professionals practicing specialist vocational rehabilitation can be a key link and support for those health care professionals delivering Levels 1 and 2 vocational rehabilitation to coordinate the IDT efforts in relation to vocational needs and goals. It is recommended that the organisations service model for vocational rehabilitation incorporates this approach into practice.

**9.** *Health care and work/education interface*

Therapists and practitioners providing Level 1 and Level 2 vocational rehabilitation will have only minimal need to communicate directly with employers and educators, but for those providing Level 3 intervention, this is an essential part of their practice. Taking work and education goals as a key focus, the specialist vocational rehabilitation practitioner is in a unique position within the IDT to operate between rehabilitation providers and the broader business and education community. By establishing and maintaining links with employers and educational agencies, improved opportunities for patients can be identified, ultimately leading to successful patient-centred vocational outcomes.

## Summary

This chapter has highlighted that within the United Kingdom, vocational rehabilitation is not universally available within health care. Access to the three levels of rehabilitation intervention following injury or illness is predominantly location dependent, and consequently can be a postcode lottery for patients nationally.

The importance of embedding vocational rehabilitation into specialist rehabilitation services has been discussed, and the Three-Level Model has been suggested as an optimum framework to support the vocational needs of rehabilitation patients. By implementing this model, it is possible to provide patients with access, at any point in their rehabilitation pathway, to vocational rehabilitation. This ensures that the service remains patient-centred, and that vocational goals are not missed but addressed at the earliest opportunity to maximise outcomes and experience. The importance of the specialist vocational rehabilitation practitioner has been discussed, and the challenges and opportunities in achieving the required skill set explained.

This chapter has sought to provide sufficient insight into the practices of vocational rehabilitation drawn from both the literature and years of practical, clinical experience within the field. However, it is acknowledged that a more in-depth exploration of the subject area is beyond the scope of a single chapter and a suggestions for reflection and references for further reading are provided at the end of this chapter. Most importantly, the aim has been to demonstrate how vocational goals are central to most patients following injury or illness, and how vocational rehabilitation can play a significant part in the completeness of a patient's recovery. Therefore, rather than viewing vocational rehabilitation as something to consider once a patient is 'better' or has returned home, it should be considered an integral element of the holistic rehabilitation of patients with complex needs.

### Reflective questions

Think about a patient you have worked with:
- How were their vocational goals explored and supported?
- Did they have Levels 1, 2, or 3 vocational rehabilitation needs?
- Which members of the IDT were involved in their vocational rehabilitation?
- Could the support they received be improved upon?
- Finally, what key points will you take away from this chapter?

# References

Allied Health Professions Federation, 2019. AHP Health and Work report. Available at: www.cop.org.uk. Accessed December 11, 2020.

British Society of Rehabilitation Medicine, 2010. Vocational Assessment and Rehabilitation for Q6 People With Long-Term Neurological Conditions: Recommendations for Best Practice. British Society of Rehabilitation Medicine. Available at: https://www.bsrm.org.uk/downloads/vr4ltncv45fl-websecure.pdf. Accessed October 9, 2021.

Council for Work and Health, 2016. Planning the Future: Implications for Occupational Health; Delivery and Training. Available at: https://www.agemanagement.cz/wp-content/uploads/2015/07/Final-Report-Planning-the-Future-Implications-for-OH-Proof-2.pdf. Accessed October 9, 2021.

Davis, K., Schoenbaum, S.C., Audet, A.M., 2005. A 2020 vision of patient-centered primary care. J. Gen. Internal Med. 20 (10), 953–957. doi:10.1111/j.1525-1497.2005.0178.x.

DH Long-term Conditions NSF Team, 2005. The national service framework for long-term conditions. Available at: https://webarchive.nationalarchives.gov.uk/ukgwa/20070305112542/; http://www.dh.gov.uk/PublicationsAndStatistics/Publications/PublicationsPolicyAndGuidance/PublicationsPolicyAndGuidanceArticle/fs/en?CONTENT_ID=4105361&chk=jl7dri. Accessed October 9, 2021.

Gail, E., 2012. Thinking Positively About Work Delivering Work Support and Vocational Rehabilitation for People With Cancer. Evaluation of the National Cancer Survivorship Initiative (NCSI) Work and Finance Workstream Vocational Rehabilitation Project. Available at: www.ncsi.org.uk/what-we-are-doing/vocational-rehabilitation/.

Kärrholm, J., et al., 2006. Effects on work resumption of a co-operation project in vocational rehabilitation. Systematic, multi-professional, client-centred and solution-oriented co-operation. Disabil. Rehab. 28 (7), 457–467. doi:10.1080/09638280500198063.

Multidisciplinary Association for Spinal Cord Injury Professionals, 2017. 'Vocational Rehabilitation Guidelines 2017 Foreword'. Available at: https://www.mascip.co.uk/wp-content/uploads/2017/11/Mascip-vocational-rehab-guidelines-Sept-2017.pdf. Accessed May 27, 2020.

NHS England, 2016. Commissioning Guidance for Rehabilitation, (04919), p. 159. Available at: https://www.england.nhs.uk/wp-content/uploads/2016/04/rehabilitation-comms-guid-16-17.pdf. Accessed December 11, 2020.

Playford, E.D. et al., 2011. 'Mapping Vocational Rehabilitation Services for People With Long Term Neurological Conditions: Summary Report', pp. 1–40. Available at: http://www.ltnc.org.uk/Researchpages/mapping_vocational_rehab.html. Accessed December 11, 2020.

Radford, K., et al., 2013. Return to work after traumatic brain injury: cohort comparison and economic evaluation. Brain Injury 27 (5), 507–520. doi:10.3109/02699052.2013.766929.

Chapter 14

# A patient's perspective

Elly Milton and Marie Milton

## Chapter outline

### Abstract

The chapter covers the personal and intimate stories of Elly and her mum Marie following Elly's life-changing stroke. They share their journey through rehabilitation, discussing the unique roles of team members, and the importance of interdisciplinary team working, communication, and person-centred care, from the patient and parent perspective. A number of reflections are presented at the end of the chapter to enhance learning and aid personal and professional development.

### Keywords

Patient perspective; Brain injury; Stroke; Rehabilitation; Family

## Introduction

Elly was 19 when she suffered a severe stroke. Because of brain swelling she required a lifesaving craniectomy (removal of a portion of skull to allow the brain to swell outwards, rather than downwards where it can compress breathing centres of the brain). She was left with a marked dysphasia (difficulty with verbal and written communication) and a dense right-sided weakness. Once acute care and early rehabilitation with the stroke team was completed, she was admitted to a Level 2 rehabilitation unit. At this stage, she required a wheelchair for mobility and assistance of two for transfers and personal care activities. With lots of hard work, sheer determination, and dedicated support from her family, Elly progressed remarkably during her 9-month hospital admission. Now back at home, her recovery and rehabilitation continue into the next phase.

Elly and her mum, Marie, have reflected on their experiences of inpatient rehabilitation on Seddon Specialist Rehabilitation Unit and have shared the following stories.

*A Practical Approach to Interdisciplinary Complex Rehabilitation.*
**DOI: https://doi.org/10.1016/B978-0-7020-8276-4.00014-X**

## Elly's story

I arrived at Seddon with mum and dad. There were lots of people in my room. They were all introducing themselves. It was very loud and felt weird. It was making my head hurt. I think it was the journey from the other hospital and the sudden change that were a bit much for me. The ward was massive! As time went on, I got used to all the different noises. There were machines beeping, room buzzers going, and people talking.

I had a chart above my bed to let the catering staff know what food I could eat. This was because I couldn't swallow to begin with, and it moved up in stages of food and drink. It started with puréed. Yuk! There was also a 'patient profile' on the wall. It was there to let people know who I was, what I liked and disliked, how to speak to me (which was slowly so I could understand) and about my family. This was really helpful as I couldn't speak at the time. The therapy team put a whiteboard in my room with the times of the different therapies and names of the therapists. There was a board in the ward with everybody's names on and session times, but as I couldn't walk, I had my own.

I had to be put in a harness for physio sessions to start with so that I could use the treadmill, but over time and a lot of hard work, I didn't need the harness and I walked with my physio lifting my foot. Her assistant kept her hands on my waist. I had a mirror in front of me so I could see my movements. I used a lot of equipment over my time in hospital for my leg; for example, a plinth, treadmill, balance bars, steps, stairs, gym ball to name a few. I used different equipment with my occupational therapist (OT) for my arm; for example, an arch, three-dimensional triangles, a mirror box, games on the computer and games like Connect 4. I also used a machine called a motomed. This was a challenge to start with, but I kept on with it and it got better.

I had to have a wheelchair that I was pushed in as my right arm and hand do not move. The therapy team came to my room when it was time for either occupational therapy, physiotherapy, or sometimes both together, and they would take me to the gym. I always had speech therapy in my room.

The nurses used to try and encourage me to go to the dining room for my meals, but I preferred to have them in my room. It was my choice, and I was never forced to eat in the dining room. I used to have my dinner with my parents in my room. They used to bring it in for me when I could eat properly. The catering staff were great. They got to know me well. They knew I had to have a plate guard so that my food didn't fall off the plate. They always put my yoghurt in a bowl as they knew I couldn't hold a pot. They even knew what lunch I would pick each day!

The therapy team always said I didn't present as a normal stroke patient, and although every stroke is different, I certainly am! I had quite a few different splints on my leg. I had a cast on it as well. It was so uncomfortable! I had a shoulder brace for a subluxation. They tried blue tape, but that really hurt and I had a reaction to it. I had a hand brace and later I had a Saebo glove too. I had a tripod walking stick and a helmet as my head needed protecting after my operation. Therapy tried a Lycra sleeve on my arm but it had the opposite effect. Botox was considered for both my arm and leg but didn't have to be used as both started to move slowly.

Speech therapy was always carried out in my room as it was quieter and I could concentrate. I remember only being able to make sounds. My therapist, Lisa, taught me how to speak again. She started teaching me how to make sounds, then names, places, pets, my job, university, and on and on until I could start joining words up and making sentences. I am right-handed but now have to write with my left. Lisa taught me to do this and to tell the time again. She was so patient with me. I used to get really tired as I had to think and find words in my head and then say them. My speech therapist would always know when I was tired.

My doctor came to see me every Friday morning to do a check-up. She came with other doctors, nurses, and students. I was the youngest on the ward at the time and had my own room.

When I wasn't in therapy I could go to group sessions, for example, arts and crafts, group psychology, and even movie nights and quizzes that my visitors could join in with. The nurses would make everybody drinks and snacks.

The therapists asked me what my goals were and helped me to achieve them. To be able to brush my teeth with my right hand again was one of them. To be able to brush my hair was another.

I went shopping with them and learned to walk and talk at the same time. I put my shopping on the belt. I said 'please' and 'thankyou' to the lady on the till. I followed a shopping list. I went Christmas shopping with my therapists. The hill in the shopping centre was huge! I climbed it though, and I got in and out of the taxi.

I was excited but nervous to go home. I was counting the days until my discharge. I felt safe in Seddon though, knowing the nurses, doctors, and therapy team were around. My main goal now I'm at home, is to live a happy and independent life. I will be forever grateful to the team at Seddon. I had such a good relationship with them. I miss them.

## Marie's story

My husband and I arrived at Seddon with our daughter Elly. After being introduced to the staff, we thought we would have a look around. It was so different to the previous ward Elly had been on. Much more relaxed. Not as hospital-like. We had a look around the dining room. It had puzzles, games, a TV, and a computer. It was used for meals, but also as a communal place where visitors could sit, group sessions were held, even quiz nights! There was a drinks machine that both patients and visitors could use free of charge. This was a blessing having previously remortgaged our house to pay for drinks and television in the hospital Elly was before! Haha. There was a television in the bays and in every room.

It was afternoon visiting time and as we entered the dining room there was a little boy crying. His dad was a patient and was telling him off. Elly was hypersensitive to noise and we could see she was starting to get distressed. I turned her wheelchair around and was heading out of the door when I literally ran a man over. It was the psychologist. He had seen what was going on and Elly's distress so came to introduce himself. He then gave us a tour of the ward. He said any of us could knock on his door at any time if we needed to talk or ask a question. It isn't just the patient who can struggle with the changes in their life, it can also have a massive impact on family and friends. So to be able to talk to someone, and not having to put on a brave face, helped a lot.

The patient's day is structured. This was important to Elly. She could not get out of bed or talk for weeks when she first arrived at Seddon, so the therapy team brought a white board into her room where they would write the time, name of the session, and names of who they were with. There was also a clock in her room so she would know when it was time for a session. The therapist would take her from her room by wheelchair and into one of the two gyms they had. Speech and language therapy was provided in her room as it was quiet so that Elly could concentrate. Her speech therapist created a 'patient profile' with Elly and put it on the wall in her room. It had details of what Elly liked and disliked, her family and friends, how to speak to her, which was slowly and directly because of her brain injury, and what she did previous to her stroke. Elly could not speak at the time, so this helped immensely with communication.

Goal-setting meetings are an important part of a patient's recovery. They are meetings that are held every 4 weeks with the patient, a doctor, a nurse, a psychologist, an OT, speech and language therapist, a physiotherapist, and the patient's family. Each person in the meeting will describe the progress made in the previous 4 weeks and will set goals for the next four. It was great being involved in the meetings. We could ask questions and would know what Elly was working towards so we could help. The therapists were so invested. They would be genuinely excited to talk about what Elly had achieved. Minutes were taken at every meeting and a copy given to the patient.

All the staff are important in the progress of a patient. Before Elly could speak again, she had a flip menu for choosing her meals, given to her by the catering staff. One of them would go through the menu for that day and she would point to what she wanted. They were so patient considering how busy they were. They knew that Elly couldn't eat a yoghurt out of its pot so always made sure it was in a bowl. She had a guard around her plate so the food couldn't fall off it. The catering staff even got to know what sandwiches she liked.

The nurses and health care assistants not only help with practical things such as showering, dressing, toilet, and baths, they get to know the patient and spend time with them. The quiz nights and movie nights are set up by them. These are great as family and visitors are included. There are two visiting times. Elly chose to just have one in the evening. This was so she could do more therapy.

Patients are allowed to go off the ward. They sign out and in on a board at the desk. There is a coffee shop in the main hospital that we went to every day. We would take Elly in her wheelchair to start with, and as she learned to walk, we would leave the wheelchair and she would walk with her stick. She even climbed the stairs!

Sometimes the physio, OT, and speech therapist would have a joint session with Elly. They would take her to the local park which she could walk to. This was so that Elly could practise walking and talking at the same time. This would take a lot of concentration and sometimes she would be so tired the next day. The team took Elly to the supermarket. She practised reaching, walking, and communicating with shop staff. This was helping to build Elly's confidence. Another trip was to do some Christmas shopping.

Visitors were so important to Elly. Elly was 19 and her friends were of the same age. Sometimes they would talk loudly and laugh lots. I remember apologising for the noise to the other patients! They said it was lovely to hear laughter and not to worry about it. After a few weeks, Elly was allowed to come home for the weekend. Before this could happen, the OT came to the house and assessed it. She ordered items that would support Elly at home, such as a commode on wheels that helped Elly to and from the toilet. As she made progress, it was replaced with a frame.

Elly was told she did not present as a 'normal' stroke patient. This was seen as a challenge for the therapy team, her OT in particular. Elly could only move the right side of her body bilaterally (when she was also using her left side) to start. Her OT had never seen this before. She researched in her own time and at weekends. She had meetings with other therapists across the country. Over the months, and plenty of hard work, the OT and physio had Elly's right side working independently.

When Elly was transferred from the stroke ward to Seddon she could not speak at all. Her speech therapist changed that! I remember the first time she said 'mum'. A word I thought I would never hear her say again. She went on to say so many more things. I sat in on quite a few sessions. I loved watching the progress. Her speech therapist would be excited when Elly would say something new. Elly had such a good relationship with her.

Physiotherapy worked with Elly's leg. I say 'worked with' because her leg used to cooperate one day and be completely uncooperative the next! Like all of her rehabilitation, her leg was a challenge. Elly was told she would probably need Botox, but within a couple of weeks it was no longer needed. The physio worked with Elly to get her walking again but also walking properly. There were so many different casts and splints trialled until the right ones were found.

We kept a diary in Elly's room so that she could look back and see her progress. Her therapists used to write a little bit about each session. Sometimes you could feel the excitement through the diary entry they had written. This used to make us feel so confident in the therapy team.

Elly was the youngest patient on the ward. As a parent it was so hard to leave her every night, but the other patients were great with her. They would call into her room for a chat or ask her if she needed anything. They would ask her to watch films in the dining room and push her there in her wheelchair. They were like a little family supporting each other. It is safe to say that if it was not for this amazing ward and it is team, my daughter would not be walking, talking, and moving as well as she does today.

Elly had her last goal-setting meeting where a date for discharge was agreed. This was to be in 4 weeks time. Elly was so excited. Within that 4 weeks the therapy team contacted the community team and invited them to Seddon to meet Elly, watch a few sessions to see how Elly presented, and to get to know her a little. This was so reassuring. There were appointments made for Elly's splints to be checked and changed if need be. An appointment was made to see Dr. Banks for a check-up. We needed to do some serious packing! I think it took 4 weeks to pack all the things she had in her room!

As happy as I was to get Elly home after 9 months in hospital and rehabilitation, I felt really nervous. We had been told by another patient that once patients are discharged into community, the level of therapy drops.

Elly was discharged on March 6, 2020. Two weeks later the country went into lockdown due to Coronavirus. This was our worst nightmare. The community team could not come. I asked for some exercises to do with Elly until they could see her which they sent. We had to be very careful as although the community team had met Elly, they had not worked with her hands on, so it was hard to choose exercises to send to us.

Anyway, we did the best we could for nearly 5 months. Elly has made improvements, and looking back, I feel it really helped being able to see how the therapists at Seddon worked. I feel I know many of the ways to help Elly hold positions and move her limbs, etc.

I was really worried about Elly's speech through lockdown. She was placed on a 12-week waiting list for community speech therapy, so Lisa, the speech therapist at Seddon, agreed to carry on with Elly so that she could continue progressing. She is now improving so much. She can actually speak in full sentences, write sentences, and tell the time again. They may only be short sentences, and she may miss or forget small words, but the improvement is huge! Through lockdown, Lisa has Skyped Elly every week with a session. She has also given her homework. This, I feel, is true commitment to her job and above.

Through all the madness of Covid, Elly has continued to make good progress. The community physiotherapist and OT are now visiting twice a week.

**Reflective questions**

- Take a moment to put yourself in Elly or Marie's position, how would you feel coming onto an unfamiliar rehabilitation unit, and how could the staff help you to settle in?

- What would be presented on your own personal 'patient profile' (or 'one page profile')? Your likes, dislikes, information about you, your family, and how best to support you.
- Elly and Marie both comment positively on some of the interventions or actions provided by the team outside of formal care. Think of a time you have provided 'extra' support or care, how may this have been interpreted/experienced by the patient and their family?
- As Marie points out, family members can also be affected by their loved one's illness/injury. How can you improve or enhance the support family members receive in your care setting?
- Think about the setting you work in, are there opportunities to enhance patient experience and how could you go about implementing changes?

Chapter 15

# Supporting the socioeconomic needs of patients and their families within the context of a complex rehabilitation setting: creating opportunities through collaboration, rehabilitation, and beyond

Claire Hendry and Erin M. Beal

## Chapter outline

**Abstract**

The aim of this chapter is to explore how socioeconomic status and disadvantages can impact negatively on an individual's overall rehabilitation. Socioeconomic factors are correlated with outcome and quality of life and therefore are an important area to assess when working in a rehabilitation setting. The chapter will aim to explore the risk factors and prevalence of injury and how it intersects with socioeconomic status. It will look at how an injury can impact the wider family network and how multiagency working can be used to effectively support people and their families post injury. Finally, it will look at a service currently practicing in the Cheshire and Merseyside Rehabilitation Network which positively supports individuals post injury.

A Practical Approach to Interdisciplinary Complex Rehabilitation.
DOI: https://doi.org/10.1016/B978-0-7020-8276-4.00015-1

**Keywords**
Socioeconomic status; Disadvantage; Socioeconomic impacts; Rehabilitation; Family;
The Life-Link Clinic; Multiagency working

## Aims

1. To describe a range of potential socio-economic needs and barriers that can be encountered by patients following complex injury or illness.
2. To understand the challenges and impacts of socio-economic factors on a patient's rehabilitation assessment, care, engagement and treatment and the wider family network.
3. To highlight the benefits of interdisciplinary team working in supporting the multi-faceted needs of patients and families.
4. To highlight potential barriers to engagement in complex rehabilitation and how interdisciplinary team working can support individuals to maximise their rehabilitation gains.

## Introduction

This chapter will consider how socioeconomic factors can intersect with disability, illness, and/or long-term health conditions, and lead to adverse long-term outcomes for patients and their families. It explores the social and economic inequalities that can be present within health care that may pose a barrier to continued patient improvement within a rehabilitation setting. The chapter also outlines a collaborative approach currently being rolled out by the Cheshire and Merseyside Rehabilitation Network, which aims to support individuals with difficulties with their socioeconomic status, during and post rehabilitation.

Let us first introduce Peter. Peter is a 37-year-old male who lives with his partner Louise and their two school-aged children in a second floor flat. They rent their home from the local housing association. Peter is employed as a lorry driver and is the sole earner in the family. Louise has a long-term health condition that impacts her ability to gain and sustain employment.

Peter presented to the rehabilitation team following a road traffic accident, where he sustained multiple physical injuries and a traumatic brain injury (TBI). He now requires a high level of support for both his physical and cognitive deficits. Peter's mood is observed to be very low post injury, and he reports high levels of anxiety and frustration at his loss of independence.

His partner Louise has confided in the team. She too is experiencing high levels of distress and feelings of hopelessness. She discloses that the family is now struggling with multiple financial pressures, as Peter is unable to return to work in the foreseeable future. She fears that the family will lose their home as they have already been threatened with eviction from the landlord. Louise is struggling to keep up with the utility bills and worries that the children's health is suffering due to an inadequate diet.

Louise reports that school has been in contact to inform her that their son is presenting with behavioural difficulties. Louise discloses that she feels very isolated and alone, she does not want to share her worries with Peter, given everything he has been through, and they have no family support in the local area.

Unfortunately, this is not an uncommon presentation within rehabilitation settings. Many individuals struggle financially post injury, which can create barriers to engagement as they begin to feel overwhelmed and stressed by external pressures, often out of their immediate control. We will consider Peter's case as we move through the chapter.

## Risk factors and prevalence

It is estimated that 1.4 million patients are seen in emergency departments every year with an acquired brain injury (ABI), with 200,000 admitted for further treatment. ABI is also the most common cause of death and disability in the United Kingdom for those aged between 1 and 40 years (NICE Clinical Guidelines, 2014). General risk factors for head injury include alcohol intoxication, age, and sex (Yates et al., 2006) with men 1.5 times more likely than women to be admitted to hospital for an ABI. However, female admissions have been rising, and there has been a 23% increase since 2005 (Headway, 2018a). Additionally, children under 5 years, who are from a socially deprived background, are at particular risk of mortality from head injury (Yates et al., 2006). The evidence base and data on prevalence rates of complex interactions of risk factors leading to neurotrauma is unfortunately scarce. The few papers which have been published report that higher rates of unemployment in the 16–24 age brackets are a risk factor predictive of higher incident rates of head injury (Tennant, 2005). Risk factors also appear to shift depending on the geographical location in the United Kingdom. It has been reported that living in a city or urban area places an individual at higher risk of a neurotrauma. However, in big cities, where individuals are more likely to commute via public transport, this can reduce the risk (e.g., in London), as driving and road traffic accidents are a large risk factor for head injury (Tennant, 2005). Data have also highlighted that children living in deprived areas are more likely to sustain severe TBIs in comparison to children from more affluent areas (Parslow et al., 2005).

The highest risk factors for ABI are felt to be; coming from a low socioeconomic status, low educational attainment, being male, and having a tendency towards risky behaviours (Her Majesty's Prison and Probation Service, 2019). Brain injuries are highly prevalent within the prison system with some reporting figures of over 60% prevalence in the prison population at any given time (Williams, 2012). Unfortunately, individuals who have a criminal record can struggle to gain meaningful employment when they are released, and there is evidence to suggest that there are links between an ABI and subsequent offending. Additionally, research also shows that those who experienced an ABI prior to the age of 12 years committed crimes significantly earlier. Furthermore, individuals' risk of subsequent ABIs increase once they have had an initial injury (Williams, 2012).

Pfeifer et al. (2011) comment that polytrauma is a 'life altering event leading to prolonged morbidity, lasting disability and immense socioeconomic burdens on the affected individual, their families and society'. They report that individuals who experience poly trauma are at an increased risk of net income loss and debt accrual. In addition, global research highlights that 53% of individuals with no fixed abode have a history of TBI, which is up to four times higher than the estimates of TBI in the general population. This population has rates of moderate to severe TBI that are 10 times higher than the general population (Stubbs et al., 2020).

Putting all of this together, current research shows that social deprivation can increase the risk of neurotrauma in childhood, leading to mortality. If the child survives the ABI however, they are then at increased risk of entering into the prison system and/or becoming homeless due to a lack of income and increasing debts. If they do enter the prison system, once released, they are less likely to gain employment as a result of a criminal record. If they are homeless, they are less likely to gain employment due to having no fixed address (along with many other factors that prevent those without a fixed abode from gaining employment). In addition to these factors, these individuals are much more likely to experience a second neurotrauma, causing further global impairment and reducing their chances of changing their circumstances. From this example, it can be seen how easily such individuals can find themselves caught in a cycle of poverty, with little to no resources available to support with breaking the cycle.

## The socioeconomic impacts of major injury and illness

For many patients embarking on their rehabilitation journey, the path forward is often unclear. Regardless of socioeconomic status, they are likely to face uncertainty regarding their future, and roles and relationships within their family and wider social networks. Many patients receiving specialist rehabilitation are confronted with the prospect of now living a different life and needing to adapt to long-term impairment following life-changing injury or illness. It is important to look beyond the immediate challenges that are faced as a result of physical and cognitive impairments, to the additional difficulties that such impairments can create and intersect with. Patients can also be faced with stressors that can impact their physical and mental health as a result of insecurity around housing, finances, and employment, in addition to potential breakdown of social relationships and isolation (Haines et al., 2019).

Patients are often unable to gain meaningful employment post brain injury and are not able to return to work, with an estimated mean of only 41% of patients, who were working prior to their injury, returning to work 1–2 years post injury (van Velzen et al., 2009). This can result in financial difficulties and increase the possibility of homelessness. There is clearly a need for vocational support to be integrated into rehabilitation models to ensure that patients return to some form of meaningful employment (see Chapter 13). Clinical guidelines stipulate that vocational rehabilitation should be provided (British Society of Rehabilitation Medicine, Royal College of Physicians, 2003). Not only would this benefit the patients, but it has also been found to be cost-effective at a societal level (Radford et al., 2013). Currently, the societal cost of ABI in terms of lost time at work and dependency on benefits is estimated to be in excess of 15 billion per annum (Parsonage, 2016).

Patients, regardless of socioeconomic status, who sustain traumatic head injuries and/or have a long-term neurological condition, have been found to experience a significantly poorer quality of life across all domains when compared to matched controls without an injury (MacHamer et al., 2013). Furthermore, the quality of life of those living in more deprived areas, combined with the impact of a disability, puts these individuals at higher risk for further health-related challenges and mental health difficulties. This is due to a widely observed association between a large range of health indicators and measures of individual socioeconomic position, such as income, educational attainment, and occupational hierarchy. These associations show that those in lower socioeconomic positions, with lower income and lower educational attainment, are more likely to have poorer physical health outcomes and poorer mental health (Braveman and Gottlieb, 2014).

With this information in mind, if we return to our case study, Peter is living in a deprived area of the Liverpool region. Liverpool has been documented as the fourth most deprived region in England and is placed third on a national scale on the domain for health and disability. It is also ranked fifth for income deprivation. Peter's flat is located in Knowsley; this area has been highlighted as the second most deprived local authority nationwide (Liverpool City Council, 2019). Therefore, prior to his injury, Peter was living in an area with fewer resources, higher rates of austerity, and was already at risk of adverse health outcomes due to these systemic factors of inequality. Returning to this environment post injury will create a unique set of barriers to his recovery that he may not face if he lived in a more affluent area. Therefore, it is imperative that socioeconomic factors be considered when developing Peter's rehabilitation goals.

Socioeconomic disadvantage can negatively impact an individual throughout their life. Within a rehabilitation setting this should be explored with Peter so that he can be given the opportunity to fully engage with his treatment and maximise his rehabilitation potential. For example, his own concerns around finances could affect his mental health, which could pose a barrier to engagement with the rehabilitation team and lead to early cessation of treatment. His level of education and reading age may affect his understanding of his condition and rehabilitation processes and communication with the team.

Socioeconomic disadvantage has many overt and covert impacts on communities and individuals that live within them. It is beyond the scope of this chapter to further explore this and it is suggested that further reading is focused on the Social Graces model (Burnham et al., 2008).

## The wider impact on family networks

Brooks (1991) coined the term 'the head injured family' to describe the impact that ABI can have on the family system. ABI, neurological conditions, and long-term health conditions can result in a wide range of cognitive and emotional difficulties that can negatively impact both the individual and their wider family network, and increase burden and stress for all (van Heugten, 2017). Jagnoor and Cameron (2014) suggest that individualised, seamless multiagency support is crucial for the treatment and care of patients and their families following major trauma and illness. It is crucial that a holistic patient-centred approach to care be implemented in order to ensure that the wider social impacts of the injury or illness are negated, or at least minimised.

Returning to Peter, the absence of his income has placed significant stress on his partner who is now concerned for the family's future, in addition to the emotional impact of the injury on each member of the family. It may be that their son is also experiencing difficult emotions, and this is presenting as behaviour that challenges in the school setting. His partner's stress levels may impact her health and her long-term health condition, and her son's education is at risk with the possibility of exclusion from school. His other child may also be suffering and require specialist support. Because of one accident and one individual's injury, there are multiple people at risk who will possibly require care; thus, potential care costs spread far beyond Peter and his injury.

ABIs have been shown to occur within a relational framework (Jumisko et al., 2007; Checklin et al., 2020). Peters relationship with his partner may suffer significantly as a result of his injury and the subsequent socioeconomic stressors they are now under. This could further impact his ability to make meaningful gains in his rehabilitation, as his attention is directed away from his rehabilitation goals to worrying about his familial relationships, debts, and financial pressures (Jumisko et al., 2007). Research has confirmed that partners of individuals with an ABI are more likely to report higher levels of burden and stress (Leathem et al., 1996; Cheng et al., 2014). Coupled with socioeconomic pressures, such as those Louise is facing, the burden is increased and can lead to breakdown of the family system. In fact, 44% of patients report breakdown of family relationships and 25% of partner relationships have ended post injury (Headway, 2018b). Children who have a parent with an ABI are at a significantly higher risk of developing post-traumatic stress symptoms (Kieffer-Kristensen et al., 2011). They are also at risk of emotional and behavioural problems if their healthy parent is experiencing stress as a result of the ill parent's injury, as this is the individual they turn to for support (Kieffer-Kristensen et al., 2013).

Unfortunately for Peter, it has also been reported that, post injury, individuals present with increased loneliness and social isolation due to breakdown of social networks (Holloway et al., 2019), with a loss in friendships being the highest breakdown of relationships post injury (Headway, 2018b). Thinking about Peter, we can assume, as the literature suggests, that his social contacts have decreased, and he is experiencing increased feelings of isolation as a direct result of his injury. The lack of expendable finances and ability to engage in activities outside the home will increase this isolation and feelings of loneliness. This may impact his mental health and subsequently feed into the negative cycle that the family have found themselves in.

This is not solely a patient-level problem, nor it is solely a problem at the family level. All the above factors will have a wider impact on health and social care support systems. These are already over stretched systems, trying to support many individuals who find themselves in similar situations to Peter across the country.

## Multiagency working; supporting the multifaceted needs of patients and families

The information presented above highlights a need for change. A recurrent theme emerging from national agendas, past and present, is the need to encapsulate the complex determinants of health inequalities and for organisations to work together to tackle such disparities (Smith et al., 1998; Marmot, 2010; Public Health England and UCL Institute of Health, 2014; Health and Social Care Act 2012, 2015; Allen et al., 2018; Group, 2018; Liverpool City Council, 2019). Woodward (2013) implores statutory organisations to familiarise themselves with local community experts and to take a broader view of the wider needs of their service users. They place the impetus on organisations to work in parallel with third sector groups, to view them as equal and valuable partners in the delivery of care. This would then allow the care of the service users to be delivered in a more comprehensive and holistic way. Henwood (2015) asserts that improvements in patient care and experience can be achieved when integrated services involve the patients in their own care. In this way, they can integrate the individual's needs and requirements into personalised treatment plans. Additionally, they should also involve experts-by-experience in service development projects to ensure that the voices of those they care for are present in the service they deliver.

The Institute of Health Equity (Allen et al., 2018) provides further evidence to support the case of services working together, and the impact that this could potentially have on health inequality. They highlight numerous examples of cross boundary working that have led to improvements in psychological wellbeing, physical health, and empowered service users. One example is the Whole Systems Data Set created by Tower Hamlets Together (Thiru et al., 2017). The Whole Systems Data Set showed that those living in the Tower Hamlets area were expected to develop poor health 10 years earlier than the average person in the United Kingdom. When looking at ill health and life expectancy, this showed that women in the area would live with 30 years of poor health and men, 25 years. This was shown to be highest in the most deprived areas, where ill health struck 12 years earlier than the more affluent areas in Tower Hamlets. Therefore, they created a partnership of local organisations, which consists of the local authority, local NHS organisations, community, and voluntary sector partners. Together they are able to look at service provision and the needs of the population in an integrated manner that stretches beyond health and social care, to education, benefits, crime, and housing. The result is a large data set of depersonalised data that highlight the wider determinates of health, and the uptake of health and social care services. They can see where to direct costs to directly benefit their community's population. This is not only of benefit to the individuals living in the Tower Hamlets area, but it is also a cost-saving initiative as they are able to target the allocation of resources.

An initiative called Life Rooms has been offered by Merseycare NHS Trust. This is a community provision that provides integrated support for individuals who are experiencing mental health difficulties. The Life Rooms project works with multiple community partners so that it can offer its patients access to education, training, welfare, and benefits advice. Users of this service have reported improvements in their confidence, wellbeing, and an increase in their employability (Harrison et al., 2017). This initiative demonstrates the importance of ensuring that the patients we see are supported in a multifaceted way in order to support their reintegration into society post injury or illness.

Another excellent example of effective multipartnership working is the Rotherham Social Prescribing Service (Dayson and Bennett, 2017). This service has adopted a multisystem partnership approach between statutory agencies and local charities to aid in the promotion of physical and mental wellbeing. This service acts as a signposting hub enabling individuals with long-term health conditions to be referred to services that meet their individual needs. Some of the services include befriending provisions to reduce social isolation, advocacy services for those that require support with decision making and impartial advice, and community lived experience groups to promote inclusion and shared experiences. An evaluation of the Social Prescribing Service highlighted numerous positive outcomes, including increased quality of life, greater satisfaction with services, and a reduction in accident and emergency admission for the population that they serve (Dayson and Bennett, 2016).

Previous survey data by the All-Party Parliamentary group on ABI reported that 93% of individuals with a brain injury found the benefits process difficult and/or unsatisfactory, over 90% agreed that the forms used to claim benefits were skewed towards physical injury and neglected cognitive difficulties, and 90% also reported that benefits assessors did not have a good insight into the challenges and impact of their ABI. In addition to this, 75% of family members did not feel that their loved one was receiving welfare benefits that met their needs (Menon, 2018). Thus, highlighting that the systems which are in place are difficult for patients and their families to access and navigate.

## The Life-Link Clinic

The authors experience is in keeping with the above and to further explore the socioeconomic issues affecting rehabilitation inpatients within the Cheshire and Merseyside Rehabilitation Network, a comprehensive inpatient staff survey was completed exploring the needs and difficulties of patients and staff. The results showed that 77% of clinicians felt that trying to support patients and their families with nonmedical issues such as housing and finances, was negatively impacting their clinical treatment sessions. These difficulties were a barrier to the clinician and the patients reaching their therapeutic goals. A subsequent survey by the first author in 2019 explored further the challenges faced by staff, patients, and family members in a rehabilitation setting, as a result of socioeconomic factors. The qualitative data presented below highlights the stark reality of the difficulties that these groups face coupled with their health needs.

One family member reflected:

*'It's a very complicated system to navigate in terms of social services, benefits and housing. It can be bewildering for people'.*

A medical staff member showed the pressure that they are under to try and ensure that their patients are getting the best level of care, but the burden that this also places on their already overstretched time:

*'On ward rounds, time and time again, patients raise issues about welfare and benefits. Trying to research these things takes up clinical time'.*

A nurse in this setting emphasised an obvious appreciation for the value of this type of support, and the impact that it would have on a patient's recovery trajectory.

*'I think it's imperative that we provide nonmedical support for our patients and their families as this can have a massive impact on mental and physical wellbeing'.*

However, a therapist also highlights the difficulties of balancing the need to provide nonmedical support to their patients, while also ensuring that they reach their rehabilitation goals:

*'Nonmedical issues can often get in the way of patients getting the best out of their treatments, which may potentially impact their outcomes'.*

It was clear from these qualitative excerpts that socioeconomic pressures, within a specialist inpatient rehabilitation setting, can impact not only on the individual and their families, but also on their clinical treatment time and outcomes. Therefore, this may lead to longer stays in hospital or rehabilitation settings and increase the financial burden on NHS services.

It may also lead to staff burnout as they compassionately attempt to support the individuals with these difficulties, which in fact lies outside of their job role description. Furthermore, some clinicians may not have had experience engaging with such services, and may therefore encounter the same difficulties that families and service users do; feelings of disempowerment due to a lack of knowledge of the system. This can lead to burnout and compassion fatigue and impact the health and wellbeing of the staff caring for and treating this population (Sodeke-Gregson et al., 2013).

Previously, the socioeconomic needs of inpatients within the Cheshire and Merseyside Rehabilitation Network were met by various organisations working in relative isolation to one another. Patients, families, and members of staff reported that this was often difficult to access and fragmented in its delivery. A newly developed provision, the Life-Link Clinic, has been created. This offers a space for multiple agencies to integrate their skills and knowledge base into the rehabilitation inpatient setting. Patients and families can access multiple services in the one place ensuring that their needs can be met without impacting on clinical time.

The Life-Link Clinic aims to assist with the holistic provision of patient-centred care to the patients and families within its remit. The overarching goal is to improve the psychological wellbeing of patients during their rehabilitation journey by alleviating the burden of navigating support systems alone. The service strives to offer a more integrated and proactive approach to supporting the socioeconomic needs of patients and to prevent socioeconomic issues affecting functional gains within rehabilitation. The Life Link service model adopts the principals of active collaborative working across the NHS to reduce health inequalities, as outlined in the Marmot Review (Marmot, 2010) and NHS England Long Term plan (Winter, 2019).

The Life-Link Clinic consists of a series of clinics facilitated by Rehabilitation Coordinators, the Local Authority, and The Brain Charity. The Brain Charity offers specialist support for both patients and families, to assist with welfare, benefits, legal advice, employment rights, education, and family advocacy services. The three agencies share their expert knowledge and skillset in order to support the nonmedical issues that patients present with post injury or illness, thus, freeing up clinical time to focus on rehabilitation goals and therapy.

Prior to the COVID-19 pandemic the clinics were held face to face to deliver advice and support in person. However, at the time of writing, the clinics are delivered once a week via a virtual platform to ensure that this vital service continues in the midst of extreme uncertainty and financial strain. Presently, all patients and family members are offered a consultation slot and are provided personalised support to access services. This may also include, but is not limited to, support with phone calls, form completion and signposting to other services. In 2018 a service evaluation by the first author showed that of those surveyed,

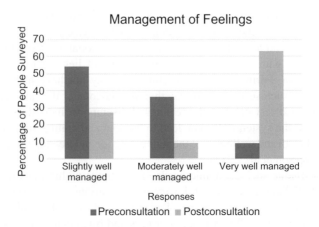

FIGURE 15.1    Responses to how feelings were managed pre- and postconsultation with the Life-Link Clinic Team.

there was a 100% satisfaction rating with the service. The qualitative feedback also indicated a self-reported significant improvement in the management and control of nonmedical issues.

The pandemic has no doubt increased inequality across society, and due to the global impact it has had on the economy, this service will be more important than ever in continuing to support the needs of individuals within rehabilitation settings. Not only is there a rise in unemployment and a record number of redundancies (ONS, 2020), there is also a rise in the prevalence of long-term health conditions as a result of contracting the virus for some individuals (Tenforde et al., 2020). The COVID-19 pandemic has also highlighted and exacerbated the systemic inequalities present within our society.

Looking at a visual representation of the service evaluation data, users of the Life-Link service reported a dramatic shift in their feelings related to their socioeconomic issues after meeting with the Life Link Team (Fig. 15.1). After the consultation meeting, over 60% felt that their nonmedical issues felt more manageable, a large rise from only 9% preconsultation. Before the meeting, nearly half of those surveyed felt that their issues were 'extremely out of control'. Post consultation over 72% reported that they either felt 'well in control' or 'very much in control' of their issues (Fig. 15.2). Before the consultation, 55% of those surveyed reported feeling 'extremely stressed and anxious' or 'moderately stressed and anxious'. Post consultation, this figure dropped to less than 20% (Fig. 15.3).

## Summary

This chapter has discussed the socioeconomic issues affecting patients undergoing rehabilitation. It has shown how a multiagency, patient-centred approach

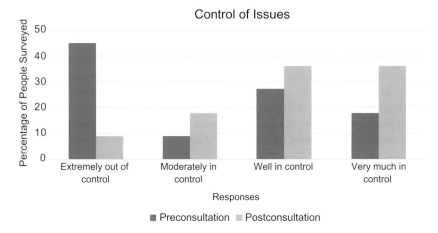

FIGURE 15.2   Responses to how in control they felt of their difficulties pre- and postconsultation with the Life-Link Clinic Team.

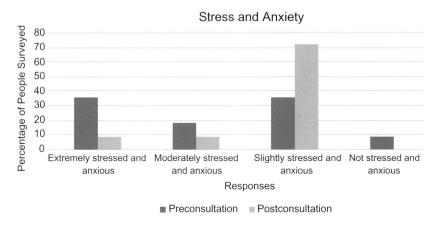

FIGURE 15.3   Responses to how stressed those surveyed felt pre- and postconsultation with the Life-Link Clinic Team.

to care can improve outcomes for patients and their family members. With appropriate exploration and support of socioeconomic factors teams can help to reduce the stress for patients, the emotional/financial burden on families, and free up clinician's time to focus on rehabilitation goals.

Returning to Peter's story, when Louise approaches the team to seek help with the wider social impacts of Peters injury, the team respectfully ask her to further explain the families struggles and needs. With Louise and Peters consent, they are referred to the Life-Link Clinic where the team further explore the difficulties that the family are facing and create a structured plan for the couple to try and alleviate some of the financial burden they are experiencing.

The couple are supported in the application for benefits which subsequently alleviates their financial difficulties. They are signposted to a children's service where their son can receive support for the difficulties he is experiencing as a result of his father's injury. This, coupled with the reduction of stress within the home, leads to an improvement in his behaviuor at school and he is no longer at risk of exclusion. Louise is also provided with education on Peter's cognitive and physical difficulties that she can share with the children to improve their understanding, patience, and subsequently their family relationships. With these pressures alleviated, Peter is engaging with his ongoing rehabilitation sessions and is making improvements across the different disciplines. His mood is improving, and he has hope and aspirations for the future.

---

### Reflective questions

- What are the main socioeconomic issues that Peter and Louise are facing?
- What are the potential outcomes for this family if these difficulties are not addressed?
- What questions would you use to assess if a patient is struggling with socioeconomic difficulties?
- Considering the services available within your region, how would you support this family?
- What are the potential benefits for Peter, his family, and the wider society, of providing support early in his rehabilitation journey?

## References

Allen, J. et al. (2018) 'Reducing Health Inequalities Through New Models of Care: A Resource for New Care Models', p. 45. Available at: www.instituteofhealthequity.org. Accessed December 11, 2020.

Braveman, P., Gottlieb, L., 2014. The social determinants of health: it's time to consider the causes of the causes. Public Health Rep. 129 (Suppl. 2), 19–31. doi:10.1177/00333549141291s206.

British Society of Rehabilitation Medicine, Royal College of Physicians, 2003. Rehabilitation Following Acquired Brain Injury. National Clinical Guidelines, vol. 81. Royal College of Physicians; British Society of Rehabilitation Medicine, London, United Kingdom, pp. 1–81.

Brooks, D.N., 1991. The head-injured family. J. Clin. Exp. Neuropsychol. 13 (1), 155–188. doi:10.1080/01688639108407214.

Burnham, J., Alvis Palma, D., Whitehouse, L., 2008. Learning as a context for differences and differences as a context for learning. J. Fam. Therapy 30 (4), 529–542. doi:10.1111/j.1467-6427.2008.00436.x.

Checklin, M., et al., 2020. What is it like to have your loved one with a severe brain injury come to rehabilitation? The experiences of significant others. Disabil. Rehab 42 (6), 788–797. doi:10.1080/09638288.2018.1510042.

Cheng, H.Y., Chair, S.Y., Chau, J.P.C., 2014. The effectiveness of psychosocial interventions for stroke family caregivers and stroke survivors: a systematic review and meta-analysis. Patient Educ. Counsel 95 (1), 30–44. doi:10.1016/j.pec.2014.01.005.

Dayson, C., Bennett, E., 2016. Evaluation of the Rotherham Mental Health Social Prescribing Pilot. Centre for Regional Economic and Social Research.

Dayson, C. and Bennett, E. (2017) 'Evaluation of the Rotherham Mental Health Social Prescribing Service 2015/16/-2016/17', Centre for Regional Economic and Social Research, p. 25. Available at: https://www4.shu.ac.uk/research/cresr/sites/shu.ac.uk/files/eval-rotherham-mental-health-social-prescribing.pdf%0Ahttp://www4.shu.ac.uk/research/cresr/sites/shu.ac.uk/files/eval-rot herham-health-social-prescribing-2015-2017.pdf. Accessed November 21, 2020.

Group, L.C.C. (2018) One Liverpool: 2018-2021. Available at: https://www.liverpoolccg.nhs.uk/media/3066/one-liverpool-plan-2.pdf. Accessed November 22, 2020.

Haines, K.L., et al., 2019. Socioeconomic status affects outcomes after severity-stratified traumatic brain injury. J. Surg. Res. 235, 131–140. doi:10.1016/j.jss.2018.09.072.

Harrison, R. et al. (2017) An evaluation of the Mersey Care Professional Advice Area. Available at: www.ljmu.ac.uk/phi. Accessed November 22, 2020.

Headway (2018a) Acquired Brain Injury: The numbers behind the hidden disability. Available at: https://www.headway.org.uk/media/7865/acquired-brain-injury-the-numbers-behind-the-hidd en-disability-2018.pdf. Accessed November 14, 2020.

Headway (2018b) 'You, me and brain injury: relationship changes after brain injury'. Available at: https://www.headway.org.uk/media/5734/relationship-changes-after-brain-injury.pdf. Accessed November 16, 2020.

Health and Social Care Act 2012 (2015) Available at: http://www.legislation.gov.uk/ukpga/2012/7/contents/enacted. Accessed November 16, 2020.

Henwood, M. (2015) Vanguard sites: new models of integration in health and social care | Social Care Network | The Guardian. Available at: https://www.theguardian.com/social-care-network/2015/mar/26/vanguard-sites-integration-health-social-care. Accessed November 22, 2020.

Her Majesty's Prison and Probation Service (2019) Traumatic brain injury in the prison population, GOV.UK. Available at: https://www.gov.uk/guidance/traumatic-brain-injury-in-the-prison-population. Accessed November 15, 2020.

Holloway, M., Orr, D., Clark-Wilson, J., 2019. Experiences of challenges and support among family members of people with acquired brain injury: a qualitative study in the UK. Brain Injury 33 (4), 401–411. doi:10.1080/02699052.2019.1566967.

Jagnoor, J., Cameron, I.D., 2014. Traumatic brain injury – support for injured people and their carers. Austral. Fam. Phys. 43 (11), 758–763. Available at: https://pubmed.ncbi.nlm.nih.gov/25393460/. Accessed November 21, 2020.

Jumisko, E., Jan Lexell, R., Söderberg, S., 2007. Living with moderate or severe traumatic brain injury the meaning of family members' experiences. J. Fam. Nurs. 13 (3), 353–369. doi:10.1177/1074840707303842.

Kieffer-Kristensen, R., Siersma, V.D., Teasdale, T.W., 2013. Family matters: parental-acquired brain injury and child functioning. NeuroRehabilitation 32 (1), 59–68. doi:10.3233/NRE-130823.

Kieffer-Kristensen, R., Teasdale, T.W., Bilenberg, N., 2011. Post-traumatic stress symptoms and psychological functioning in children of parents with acquired brain injury. Brain Injury 25 (7–8), 752–760. doi:10.3109/02699052.2011.579933.

Leathem, J., Heath, E., Woolley, C., 1996. 'Relatives' perceptions of role change, social support and stress after traumatic brain injury. Brain Injury 10 (1), 27–38. doi:10.1080/026990596124692.

Liverpool City Council (2019) 'The Index of Multiple Deprivation 2010 a Liverpool Analysis', pp. 1–42. Available at: https://www.gov.uk/government/statistics/english-indices-of-deprivation-2019. Accessed November 21, 2020.

MacHamer, J., Temkin, N., Dikmen, S., 2013. Health-related quality of life in traumatic brain injury: is a proxy report necessary? J. Neurotrauma 30 (22), 1845–1851. doi:10.1089/neu.2013.2920.

Marmot, M. (2010) Fair Society, Healthy Lives. The Marmort Review, Executive Summary. Available at: http://www.instituteofhealthequity.org/resources-reports/fair-society-healthy-lives-the-marmot-review/fair-society-healthy-lives-exec-summary-pdf.pdf. Accessed November 22, 2020.

Menon, D.K. (2018) Time for Change Acquired Brain Injury and Neurorehabilitation Time for Change Education Neurorehabilitation Criminal Justice Sport-Related Concussion Welfare Benefits System Time for Change Executive Editor. Available at: www.ukabif.org.ukwww.ukabif.org.uk. Accessed November 14, 2020.

National Institute for Health and Care Excellence (UK) (2019) NICE Clinical Guidelines, N. 176. Head injury: assessment and early management Clinical guideline. Available at: www.nice.org.uk/guidance/cg176. Accessed September 14, 2020.

ONS, 2020. Labour Market Overview, UK. Office for National Statistics.

Parslow, R.C., et al., 2005. Epidemiology of traumatic brain injury in children receiving intensive care in the UK. Arch. Dis. Childhood 90 (11), 1182–1187. doi:10.1136/adc.2005.072405.

Parsonage, M. (2016) 'Traumatic brain injury and offending: an economic analysis', p. 30. Available at: https://www.centreformentalhealth.org.uk/sites/default/files/2018-09/Traumatic_brain_injury_and_offending.pdf. Accessed December 15, 2020.

Pfeifer, R., et al., 2011. Socio-economic outcome after blunt orthopaedic trauma: implications on injury prevention. Patient Saf. Surg. 5 (1), 9. doi:10.1186/1754-9493-5-9.

Public Health England and UCL Institute of Health (2014) Local action on health inequalities. Available at: www.instituteofhealthequity.org. Accessed November 22, 2020.

Radford, K., et al., 2013. Return to work after traumatic brain injury: cohort comparison and economic evaluation. Brain Injury 27 (5), 507–520. doi:10.3109/02699052.2013.766929.

Smith, G.D., Morris, J.N., Shaw, M., 1998. The independent inquiry into inequalities in health. Br. Med. J. 317 (7171), 1465–1466. doi:10.1136/bmj.317.7171.1465.

Sodeke-Gregson, E.A., Holttum, S., Billings, J., 2013. Compassion satisfaction, burnout, and secondary traumatic stress in UK therapists who work with adult trauma clients. Eur. J. Psychotraumatol. 4 (Suppl.), 21869. doi:10.3402/ejpt.v4i0.21869.

Stubbs, J.L., et al., 2020. Traumatic brain injury in homeless and marginally housed individuals: a systematic review and meta-analysis. Lancet Public Health 5 (1), e19–e32. doi:10.1016/S2468-2667(19)30188-4.

Tenforde, M.W., et al., 2020. Symptom duration and risk factors for delayed return to usual health among outpatients with COVID-19 in a Multistate Health Care Systems Network—United States, March–June 2020. MMWR Morbid. Mortality Wkly. Rep. 69 (30), 993–998. doi:10.15585/mmwr.mm6930e1.

Tennant, A., 2005. Admission to hospital following head injury in England: incidence and socio-economic associations. BMC Public Health 5 (1), 21. doi:10.1186/1471-2458-5-21.

Thiru, K., Goldblatt, P. and Hogarth, S. (2017) Guide to the Creation of a Whole Systems Data Set. Available at: http://www.instituteofhealthequity.org/file-manager/NHSE_CASE_STUDIES/a-guide-to-creating-a-whole-system-dataset-tower-hamlets-together-2018.pdf. Accessed November 22, 2020.

van Heugten, C.M. (2017) 'Adults with non-progressive brain injury b). Stroke', In Wilson, B., Winegardner, J., Van Heugten, C.M., Ownsworth, T. (Eds.), Neuropsychological Rehabilitation: The International Handbook. Abingdon, Oxon: Routledge, pp. 65–69.

van Velzen, J.M. et al. (2009) 'How many people return to work after acquired brain injury?: A systematic review', Brain Injury, pp. 473–488. doi: 10.1080/02699050902970737

Williams, H. (2012) 'Repairing shattered lives'. Available at: https://barrowcadbury.org.uk/wp-content/uploads/2012/11/Repairing-Shattered-Lives_Report.pdf. Accessed November 15, 2020.

Winter, G., 2019. The NHS long term plan. J. Prescribing Pract. 1 (3), 114. doi:10.12968/jprp.2019.1.3.114, –114.

Woodward, P. (2013) How the voluntary sector can save an overstretched NHS | Healthcare Professionals Network | The Guardian. Available at: https://www.theguardian.com/healthcare-network/2013/feb/25/how-voluntary-sector-can-save-nhs. Accessed November 22, 2020.

Yates, P.J., et al., 2006. An epidemiological study of head injuries in a UK population attending an emergency department. J. Neurol. Neurosurg. Psychiatry 77 (5), 699–701. doi:10.1136/jnnp.2005.081901.

Chapter 16

# Conclusion

Cara Pelser, Angela Harrison, Ganesh Bavikatte, and Helen Banks

Firstly, thank you for taking the time to read and engage with the book, or as many chapters as you felt necessary for your personal development or special interest. By assembling 15 chapters, comprehensively written by authors who are currently practising in the field, the aim of the book was to provide a valuable insight into the holistic delivery of complex, patient-centred, rehabilitation.

As editors and authors, we hope that you have learnt something new, refreshed your knowledge, or intensified your passion for exploring the field of complex rehabilitation further. Each chapter set out to cover a set of aims and objectives pertinent to true interdisciplinary team (IDT) working. We hope each chapter gave you the opportunity to step back and reflect on your practice, your role, and your personal and professional values. Going forward, our aim is that this book encourages collaboration, communication, and shared goal setting with colleagues and like-minded individuals.

Working in complex rehabilitation requires teamwork. Knowing and understanding the roles and responsibilities of the people around you will only serve to enhance your practice, and most importantly, the patient experience. The patient is at the heart of the work we do, the decisions we make and the reasons we all decided to work within health care in the first place. Elly and her mum, Marie, in Chapter 14, shared their experience of IDT working and how they felt supported and encouraged by everyone around them, thus demonstrating the importance and effectiveness of teamwork and person centred care. The team working with Elly and her family ensured that she had the best possible chance of returning to her previous role, responsibilities and activities, and were willing to go the extra mile to make this possible.

Each patient has different and diverse biopsychosocial rehabilitation needs; from memory impairment or a communication disorder, to difficulties with movement and coordination, swallow or navigating a return to work. Complex rehabilitation is therefore about working together, with the patient and family/carers, to ensure that the rehabilitation experience is focused on meaningful,

A Practical Approach to Interdisciplinary Complex Rehabilitation.
DOI: https://doi.org/10.1016/B978-0-7020-8276-4.00016-3

realistic, idiosyncratic, and often dynamic, patient goals. As an IDT, it is therefore our role and responsibility to collectively apply our knowledge and skills to the understanding and treatment of individuals, to optimise outcomes in terms of health, independence, and daily functioning.

We hope this book makes a unique and substantial contribution to the field of complex rehabilitation.

# Index

Page numbers followed by "*f*" and "*t*" indicate, figures and tables respectively.